BEITRÄGE ZUR ERNÄHRUNGSWISSENSCHAFT

BEITRÄGE ZUR ERNÄHRUNGSWISSENSCHAFT

Herausgegeben von

W. DIEMAIR **J. KURPIANOFF** **K. LANG** **C. H. MELLINGHOFF**
Frankfurt a. M. Karlsruhe Mainz Wuppertal

Band 6

NUTRITION AND CARIES

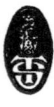

DARMSTADT 1961

DR. DIETRICH STEINKOPFF VERLAG

NUTRITION AND CARIES

Editor:

B.C.P. JANSEN

Emeritus Professor of Physiological Chemistry at the Amsterdam University
Former Head of The Netherlands Institute of Nutrition

With Contributions from

Dr. L. M. DALDERUP ∕ Amsterdam, Prof. Dr. B.C.P. JANSEN ∕ Amsterdam,
Dr. R. LUYKEN ∕ Utrecht, and Dr. M. NEDERVEEN ∕ FENENGA ∕ Amstelveen

With 3 Tables

DARMSTADT 1961

DR. DIETRICH STEINKOPFF VERLAG

ISBN-13: 978-3-642-87678-3   ISBN-13: 978-3-642-87676-9
DOI: 10.1007/978-3-642-87676-9

Copyright 1961 by Dr. Dietrich Steinkopff, Darmstadt
Softcover reprint of the hardcover 1st edition 1961

Zweck und Ziel der Sammlung

Angesichts der wachsenden Bedeutung der Ernährungswissenschaft als Grenzgebiet zwischen Medizin, Physiologie, physiologischer Chemie, Chemie und chemischer Technologie entstand das Bedürfnis nach einem wirklich *wissenschaftlichen Publikationsforum* für die Arbeitsergebnisse dieses Forschungszweiges. Es gilt, die Erkenntnisse und Erfahrungen *aller* unmittelbar und mittelbar beteiligten Teildisziplinen zu sammeln.

Um dafür einen gemeinsamen Rahmen zu bieten, wurde die Sammlung „Beiträge zur Ernährungswissenschaft" geschaffen. Der Plan für diese Sammlung besteht schon seit längerer Zeit, konnte aber zunächst infolge der unübersichtlichen Nachkriegsverhältnisse nicht verwirklicht werden. Sowohl knapp gefaßte, richtungweisende Forschungsberichte und Monographien über spezielle Probleme als auch zusammenfassende Darstellungen eines geschlossenen größeren Gebietes sollen im Rahmen der Sammlung erscheinen. Die Existenz eines solchen Publikationsforums soll auch anregend auf die literarische Behandlung wissenschaftlicher Ernährungsprobleme wirken.

Die Sammlung umfaßt also Beiträge aus *allen Zweigen der Ernährungswissenschaft*, von der *Physiologie* und *Klinik* (einschließlich Diätetik, Säuglings- und Krankenernährung), *Chemie* (insbesondere in ihren Zweigen Agrikulturchemie, Lebensmittelchemie, physiologische Chemie), *chemischen Technologie*, *Landwirtschaftswissenschaft* (besonders angewandte Boden-, Dünger- und Fütterungslehre, Züchtung) bis zur *Veterinärmedizin* und zu den *Ingenieurwissenschaften* (Haltbarmachung durch Gefrieren, Sterilisieren; Trocknen und Verpacken) sowie schließlich zu Problemen der Verpflegungs- und Küchenorganisation. Die Darstellung soll jeweils knapp, verständlich und anregend sein, ohne den Boden der Wissenschaftlichkeit zu verlassen.

Dem Charakter der Sammlung gemäß wird erstrebt, nach und nach das gesamte Gebiet der Ernährungswissenschaft den neuesten wissenschaftlichen Erkenntnissen entsprechend darzustellen.

Frühjahr 1957

HERAUSGEBER UND VERLAG

Preface

For many years we have known that dental caries is one of the most common diseases of mankind. Only few people have sound teeth till the end of life. Formerly we thought that the only possibility to keep our teeth in good state was to go to the dentist regularly. Since we know how complicated our nutrition is we know too that we have to regard the composition of our food as a principal factor influencing the state of our teeth. The trace-elements e. g. play an important role.

Studies with tracers during the last decades have shown that the minerals are metabolized very actively by living organisms. Thus research in our laboratory, together with Prof. Sizoo and Prof. Dols, has demonstrated that intravenously injected radio-active phosphorus has disappeared from the blood already half an hour after injection. Even the hard dental substance participates in this active metabolism.

I think that the work of Lady Mellanby, years ago, proves very well the influence of nutrition on the health of our teeth. Lady Mellanby investigated the teeth of the many dogs used by her husband in rickets research. She found a remarkable hypoplasia of the teeth. I think indeed that the deficiency of vitamin D is the cause of hypoplasia in young dogs. Another question is whether vitamin D deficiency is connected with caries. Lady Mellanby found with experiments in boarding-schools that children with extra vitamin D had less caries than the children without vitamin D. Nevertheless there were some new cases of caries in the former group.

Another component of our food, vitamin A, influences the internal structure of the teeth as has been shown by Wolbach and Howe and by King.

These examples showing the relation between nutrition and the health of our teeth can be amplified by many others. The former work on the influence of nutrition on dental caries is already fully reviewed in the book „A survey of the literature of dental caries" by the National Research Council (Washington, D. C. 1952). Now I have the pleasure to introduce the recent work of three of my collaborators in the Netherlands Institute of Nutrition, Amsterdam.

Dr. R. Luyken, M. D. Amsterdam, has worked for years on nutritional problems and has several times carried out a survey in the Far East and in the Carribean Area.

Mrs. NEDERVEEN-FENENGA, M. D. Amsterdam, D. D. S. Utrecht, formerly head of the Dental School Service in Amsterdam.

Dr. L. M. DALDERUP, M. D. Amsterdam, Ph. D. Amsterdam, who carried out extensive work for many years on experimental caries laboratory animals and developed an ingenious new method for evaluation initial caries lesions.

Spring 1961   B. C. P. JANSEN

Contents

I. Aetiology of Dental Caries

A few Short Remarks

For many years much has already been written about the causes of dental caries but, still little is actually known about the how, when, why, and the exact where of the onset of the carious process.

Naturally, theories have been formulated to explain the attack. There are, however, only a few fundamentally different ones, probably due to the impression of apparent simplicity of the dental tissue. The most outstanding characteristic of the structure of this tissue is its extraordinarily high mineral content. It is not surprising, therefore, that decomposition of these minerals was once looked upon as the main aspect of carious processes.

The first and oldest theory is the one set up by W. D. MILLER (1), the chemicoparasitic theory, commonly misinterpreted as the "acidogenic theory", indicating that the primary cause was thought to be an attack by acids. MILLER himself was of the opinion that all acid producing bacteria in the mouth should be held responsible. Later investigators focussed interest on the lactobacillus, which produces large quantities of lactic acid, and they nearly forgot other bacteria possibly playing a rôle. This is not so strange as it seems, since lactobacillus is always present in the flora of the mouth and generally in larger quantities if there are many carious lesions. In fact, an attack by acids of such a highly mineralized tissue as dental enamel necessarily seems to be important in the production of dental caries. However, it is not certain „a priori" that the initial attack must be made by acid(s). Moreover, acids by themselves, in food or beverages, or factory dust, do give erosion or attrition but no caries of the teeth. Since enamel has a framework of organic material in which the enamel rods are built in, an attack through the organic part might also play a rôle [BÖDECKER (2)], and it is as plausible, theoretically, to assume a proteolytic process as the initial stage [GOTTLIEB (3), PINCUS (4)]. However, it proved to be very difficult to provide conclusive evidence that proteolytic processes alone can provoke caries; some acid seemed to be necessary.

Later on, in 1949, PINCUS (5) suggested that a sulphatase produced by a type of gram-negative bacillus in the mouth might play an important role. The sulphatase should attack mucoproteins, as a result of which sulphuric acid is released, which could attack on its turn the mineral part of the teeth. However, without previous hydrolysis of the mucoproteins the enzyme seemed to be inactive.

GOTTLIEB (3,6) believed that the lamellae of the enamel constituted the access to the deeper parts of the tooth. As a matter of fact, caries attack does not necessarily mean that the whole layer of the enamel is invaded over a particular area. It is possible and does occur, but the lamellae may also form a path into the inner structures of the tooth. Although narrow, the lamellae seem to offer bacteria ample opportunity to penetrate deeply. Notably the dentino-enamel junction may be affected over a wide area without severe destruction of the overlying enamel. The dentine may be attacked later on and also the enamel could come to suffer from attack from the inside. Staining reactions in rats have demonstrated that these processes may occur in all graduations and combinations. Moreover, they depend upon the diet given. In the initial stages, the lesions in rats – a special study has been made of those in the fissures – are very similar to the picture observed in man [NEDERVEEN-FENENGA and DALDERUP (7)].

Obviously, the matter is very complicated because it appeared that intact enamel is permeable to a number of substances, including iodine, calcium, phosphorus, dyes, glucose and tetanus toxine [BARTELSTONE (8), SOGNNAES and SHAW (9), JANSEN and VISSER (10), BERGGREN and HEDSTRÖM (11)].

It is evident that the substrate for the bacteria involved in the carious attack is formed by dental deposits and food debris. Especially sugar and carbohydrates are regarded as injurious, and this is independent of the fact whether acidogenic, proteolytic or perhaps sulphatase reactions take place initially. The harmful substances which are produced by the oral flora could than attack the dental tissue and thus permit a bacterial invasion into this tissue. The presence of bacteria seems to be imperative for a carious attack, as was observed in experiments on germfree animals [ORLAND, BLANEY and many others (12)] and revealed by studies on the effects of antibiotics [STEPHEN, FITZGERALD and McCLURE et al. (13); STEPHEN, HARRIS and FITZGERALD (14); FITZGERALD (15)]. On the other hand, the absence of bacteria is not an absolute condition for the absence or prevention of dental caries.

However, for all three theories the findings of many experiments carried out 'in vivo' and 'in vitro' by a great many investigators could not be brought completely in concordance with the view of a prevalence of one of other mode of initial attack. It is therefore that the recent theory claimed by SCHATZ and MARTIN (16. 17) and by SCHATZ, KARLSON, MARTIN and SCHATZ (18) is so very attractive. The principles explained by these authors describing caries as a process of chelation (derived from the Greek word ,chela', which means claw or pincer) or of proteolysis-chelation unite the two processes – proteolytic and acidogenic – together. Both types of attack do occur together and simultaneously instead of an independent attack by either of these alone. Chelating agents, generally can combine with a metal to form stable complexes in which the metal is non-ionized. The resulting complexes have a ring structure. The water-soluble complexes can readily be carried off from all surfaces which come to suffer from an chelation attack.

On every occasion the energetically more stable ring structure will be formed, and thus here also competition of a number of substances capable of chelation must play an enormous role. The chelation principle is very common in biological enzymatic processes. Haemoglobin, for instance, can be considered as such a chelated substance containing iron in the ring. The same applies to chlorophyl, in which the metal bound is magnesium. It is known now, that many products, including lactic acid, as well as the intermediate metabolites of for instance the Krebs cycle, have a chelating activity. But chelation is not at all limited to these products. Lipids, for instance, can chelate as well. It is known that a synthetic chelating agent, E. D. T. A. (aethylene-diamine-tetra-acetic acid, also called complexon or versene) promotes dental caries in rats if it is added to the food [STEPHEN and HARRIS (19)]. However, when it is administered by stomach tube, it has little if any effect [SHAW and GUPTA (20)]. In concordance with the abovementioned opinion as regards competition, not all E. D. T. A. salts have a caries-stimulating or have an equal serious effect [HENDERSHOT and FORSAITH (21)]. The disodium salt, the magnesium salt and the cobalt salt for instance increase dental caries three- or fourfold, whereas the zinc and nickel salts produce a reduction of dental caries to one-fourth up to one-tenth as compared with the controls. The calcium, manganese, iron and copper salts have little effect.

Furthermore, according to SCHATZ, KARLSON, and MARTIN (22), the enamel minerals $Ca_3(PO_4)_2$, $CaCO_3$, as well as the trace elements, stimulate the keratinolysis by bacteria and, on the other hand, keratinolysis contributes to the dissolution of the enamel apatite. The greater part of the organic matrix of enamel is keratin*); in addition, there are small amounts of mucopolysaccharides and lipids. The break-down of the matrix constituents releases chelating agents, and so the mineral part is attacked simultaneously, Moreover, the chelating

---

*) It has recently been claimed that the enamel protein shows a greater resemblance to collagen than to keratin, based on its amino acid composition [GELLER (23)].

substances need not originate from the dental matrix but may come from dental deposits.

In principle there is no difference according to SCHATZ et al. from the mechanism which comes into play in cases of pathological bone resorption, the root resorption of normal deciduous teeth, some diseases in the calcareous shells of crabs and molluscs, and even from the solubilization of rock phosphate (apatite) fertilizers in alkaline and neutral soils. SCHATZ, KARLSON and MARTIN (22) strongly emphasize that acids need not absolutely be the only or even the main factor in these processes.

So far as dental caries is concerned, the oral flora seems both to be capable of and necessary to start this process. Consequently, the microorganisms, enzymes and metabolites are extremely important. SCHATZ et al. demonstrated especially the importance of the proteolysis-chelation combination, and used not only enamel and dentin (human and rat) but also hair (keratin) in their experiments. Recently PEPPER, HUGHSTON, EARLE and BINCKLEY (24) demonstrated that enzymatic depolimerization of chondroitin-sulphate by oral streptococci, releasing hexosamine, is possible. On a substrate of cleaned and pulverized cattle teeth, streptococci were even more active than on commercial chondroitin-sulphate.

According to EGGERS LURA (25), three chemical reactions taking place in proteolysis-chelation processes are known to be activated by sucrose and glucose. These reactions are the following: keratinolysis, the activity of bacterial phosphatases, and also the chelation mechanism of the metal complex itself. The new conceptions on the initial carious attack certainly have consequences for the tentative prevention of caries. So far, this prophylaxis has mainly been directed to the prevention of acid formation. However, the aim should now be to prevent the formation of products which are capable of chelating (substances from the teeth) or which activate the chelating process. In this way, EGGERS LURA came to the conclusion that attempts should be made to have all food debris oxidized by the oral flora to CO_2 and H_2O as thoroughly and as early as possible, so as to ensure that no accumulation of intermediate products capable of tooth destruction occurs. Practical procedures to reach this aim would be diluting the food by masticating thoroughly and by drinking water, beer or wine after meals, and, of course, by limiting eating between meals. In this respect, it is of special importance that sticky food be avoided. For the present this only means in practice that the same measures should be taken as those recommended for the elimination of acids.

Amplifying these ideas and emphasizing their value, are the observations of BRAMSTEDT, KRÖNCKE and NAUJOKS (26), who demonstrated that fluorine concentrations in the saliva, such as do occur on fluoridation of drinking-water (M 10^{-4}, 10^{-5}, 10^{-6}), activate the anaerobic glucose desintegration by a number of bacteria which occur in the oral flora of man. Moreover, the fluoride-treated tooth is better resistant to chelation attack than a non-treated tooth.

In addition, the important role which certain metals, in appropriate doses, and appropriate salts, seem to play, such as for instance Tin, Vanadium, Molybdenum and Strontium (in a favourable manner) and Selenium and Cadmium (in an unfavourable manner), might be related to their chelating capacities, thus chelating constants, or to possible inhibitory or activating influences or the chelation process. In the same manner, their toxic action – already present in very small doses – could be attributed to these same properties. But other modes of action may also play a role.

It is impossible to give more than a very brief impression of the work done, all the facts known and, of all the problems that have been encountered in the study of dental caries. A good deal about the work done before 1956 may be found in the following excellent surveys of problems concerning dental caries: „Survey of the Literature on Dental Caries" (27), „Advances in Experimental Caries Research" (28), and in the survey composed by LAMMERS and HAFER (29).

II. Histology of Normal and Carious Dental Tissue

A. Introduction

As a result of refinements and renovations of investigation techniques our knowledge of the histology of dental tissue has considerably been enriched in recent years. This advance includes both normal and pathological histology. As far as the latter is concerned dental caries in particular is implied.

Investigation into the embryological development of dental tissue has also revealed a number of enlightening facts.

The methods of investigation described below have been regularly used in recent years.

1. Simple Microscopy

Advances have principally occurred by improvements in staining techniques, by means of using thinner cuts and by the altered methods for decalcification. Thinner sections are obtained mainly by an improvement in the sectioning apparatus.

These principally technical advances have not much changed the insight into the histology of dental tissue and discussion of this subject will not be considered any further in this chapter.

2. Ground Sections

Ground sections, that are still used fairly often, were further investigated in recent years. Attention is particularly directed to the investigation after removal of the organic material from the dental tissue.

3. Electron Microscopy

This has proved to be an important acquisition. However one should be somewhat reserved in interpreting the results of the pictures observed.

Another difficulty is that even when it is possible to cut sections to a thickness of 0.005 μ with an ultramicrotome one can only photograph sections that do not evaporate any more in the vacuum, that must be applied in the electron microscope. These sections must thus be completely dehydrated when they are introduced into the electron microscope. This can be amplified to a certain extent by making replicas. In this way the surface of the tissue can be examined and many details about the surface of the enamel and dentine are revealed.

4. Polarization Microscopy

This method is still often used to supplement the methods of investigation mentioned above.

5. Radioactive Isotopes

A better insight into the metabolism of enamel and dentine is obtained by the use of radio isotopes. It is possible to follow the fluid current in the dental tissue and to observe the intake and delivery of various atoms. We will summarize the most recent data under the following subdivisions.

B. Data Obtained During the Investigation of Odontogenesis

In animals the development of hard dental tissue can be followed quite well to the time when decalcification of these tissues commences. Until then very thin sections can be made of the tissue to be investigated without previously decalcifying it. The latter procedure gives more possibilities of introducing tissue changes.

It was principally LEFKOWITZ, BODECKER and MARDFIN (30) who studied the odontogenesis of rat molars. They made frontal and sagittal sections of the molars of rat embryos so that a dimensional picture was obtained. Mainly with the intention of being able to study better the pathological lesions at a later date they followed the changes taking place in the formation of normal enamel and dentine from day to day. They described the first mucosal changes at the site where the teeth must arise later and established that this occurred on the 13th day of embryo life. Their investigation extended from the 13th embryonal day until the birth of the animal. In this investigation it is striking that is was found that in the rat the outermost enamel epithelium does not remain. Many blood vessels arise at this site. Moreover the reticulum stellare only remains a few days. They find that differentiation to ameloblasts first occurs after the formation of dentine has commenced and thus arrive at the same conclusion as many other investigators before them.

It is remarkable that no data are available in the recent literature about the so-called basal membrane. During the development of the dental tissue we can observe that the ameloblasts are separated from the odontoblasts by the basal membrane, which however disappears when the hard dental tissue forms. It is supposed that this membrane is important for the formation of enamel and dentine that will take place later but the role that it plays here as well as the composition of the membrane itself are equally vague. Possibly a further investigation on these points by means of the electron microscope can reveal with more certainty just what role it does play. In 1955 MYERS (31) further investigated the formation of the enamel making use of radioactive calcium. It is generally assumed that this takes place in 2 successive stages, namely

1) Matrix formation i. e. the organic phase and

2) Calcification i. e. the inorganic phase.

The investigation was intended to ascertain how the calcium reached the matrix during calcification. Both by radio-autography and X-ray photographs it can be demonstrated that the matrix receives its calcium from outside. Moreover it appeared that calcification of the enamel does not reach its maximum intensity immediately but that the enamel layers nearest to the dentine, which are the first to calcify, still take up radioactive calcium for quite a long time afterwards whilst they also absorb very many soft X-rays. This ripening of the enamel evidently extends over the whole period between the completion of the matrix and the eruption of the teeth.

C. Data Concerning Completed Dental Tissue

1. Enamel

For a long time it was supposed that enamel, in contrary to the dentine, demonstrated no single form of metabolism. Further investigations during the last 10 years threw doubt upon the accuracy of this point of view. After investigating enamel with radioactive materials both BERGGREN (32) in 1947, BARTLESTONE (33) in 1950 and WAINWRIGHT (34) in 1954 came to the conclusion that some metabolism does take place in enamel. In 1947 BERGGREN e. g. could demonstrate by means of radioactive phosphorus that enamel both in a centrifugal as well as in a centripetal direction is permeable to phosphorus.

A number of investigations has been carried out into the structure of the enamel recently. The publication of LOSEE (36) concerning the so-called lamellae is first worth mentioning. These structures originally described by BODECKER (37) in 1906 were only found in completed enamel. Under the microscope he saw the lamellae as stripes in the enamel, which ran from the dentino-enamel junction to the outermost layers of the enamel. He thought they must have originated from organic material, basing these ideas on the reactions with certain dyes. Since then many ideas and investigations have been directed to find out if these lamellae actually exist and if so, what is their function. LOSEE (36) described cut sections made of human teeth. These sections were exposed to 1.2-diaminoethane steam which is a substance that extracts organic material from the sections. They were then viewed by means of polarized light. Coloured photographs demonstrated that after this operation a number of microlamellae become visible and have a remarkably similar structure to the lamellae of BODECKER. As a result of this investigation, and the many publications that have appeared on this subject, the existence of the enamel lamellae can definitely be assumed to exist. Their function however is not yet elucidated notwithstanding a number of attempts carried out in this direction.

The RETZIUS stripes in the enamel also remain a debatable point. In 1957 PANTKE (38) presented a review of the many opinions that exist about theses stripes. By means of a replica technique he could demonstrate that these stripes also occur in the enamel of milk teeth formed pre- and postnatally. In 1955 TAKUMA (39), on studying decalcified enamel, found that the enamel prismata are not surrounded by the organic matrix on all sides. On some enamel prismata they found namely that the matrix was interrupted on one side and considered that this sign was due to the fact that compression and contraction of the matrix took place during decalcification. Using electron microscopy they presented a detailed description in their article of the fixation methods, the material used for imbedding and of the ultramicrotome. A further confirmation of their conclusions however is desired.

Many investigators were fascinated by the membrane that is found on the surface of the enamel after the teeth have fully grown, the socalled membrane of NASMYTH. GOTTLIEB (6) distinguished 2 layers in it: one, a keratine layer, directly adjacent to the enamel which is the most recent product of the ameloblasts and, another outside this which is a layer of degenerated ameloblasts. MAXIMOW and BLOOM (40) also describe 2 membranes in their book as being the most recent product of the activity of the ameloblasts and point out that these membranes consist of mucoprotein. It is often assumed that these membranes cannot be observed any more at a later age due to their being ground down. KLEES et al. (41) on the contrary presented a detailed review of the literature about the membrane of Nasmyth and stated that the membrane possessed regenerative properties so that after it is ground down together with the surface layer of the enamel a new membrane can be rapidly formed. This opinion, that was first described by these investigators, cannot however be regarded as a generally assumed fact.

GUSTAFSON (42) studied the histological changes of human enamel in initiating caries. The investigation was aimed especially at the decalcified spots in the enamel that amongst others were studied with the polarization microscope. He described 5 layers in the enamel in caries. From the pulp to the enamel these are recognized as follows.

a) A layer characterized by a high mineral content.
b) A layer in which the calcium salts can be dissolved.
c) A zone with a raised calcium content.
d) A zone in which calcium salts are dissolved and the organic material is affected.
e) A layer where the enamel is destroyed.

GUSTAFSON in this extensive article describes moreover that fissure caries does not commence at the bottom at the fissure but that it first commences actually at the entrance to the fissure. This is in contrary to the many publications about the subject where commencing caries is observed at the bottom of the fissure.

The opinions concerning initiating caries still remain divergent. In 1860 LEBER and ROTTENSTEIN (43) thought that dental caries is caused by the action of acids on the enamel of teeth and molars. After this in 1890, MILLER (44) developed his chemico-parasitie theory which is a theoretical view that up to the present day cannot be completely established or refuted by any scientific worker. Many investigators, amongst whom are those of the „Michigan Workshop", accept the caries theory of MILLER and base the purpose of their investigation on this theory. MILLER considers that the acid-producing bacteria, that are fo und on the surface of the teeth, are responsible for the production of acids. The resulting decalcification of the enamel forms the first stage of caries.

BODECKER (45) thought that the initial stage of caries was due to the action of proteolytic-working bacteria.

VON BARTHELD (46) again pointed out that caries of the enamel begins as a white discoloration but, without affecting the characteristic structure on the surface nor the internal structure of the enamel. Macroscopically the affected region appears as a chalky-white, opaque mass, in contrary to the remaining transparent tissue. It is easy to scratch it with a probe. Microscopically however the picture is only altered in so far that in general the structure of the enamel has become more distinct whilst the opaque tissue is yellowish in colour when viewed by transmitted light. It contains less calcium salts. This can be regarded as a result of a slow decalcification, activated by the acid metabolic products of certain oral bacteria. VON BARTHELD pointed out that the weak point in the theory of Miller is that the acids formed affect the enamel as soon the pH falls below a certain level. Furthermore he stated in his investigation that the occurrence of white patches in the enamel in early caries can be explained as a result of the presence of positive protein ions on the surface and not necessarily the presence of free acids.

More and more in the literature one sees that the initiation of the carious process is sought for in this direction. A large number of experts on the subject of caries is convinced that in a carious process decalcification first occurs followed by proteolysis. However there still remain a few experts who consider that proteolysis plays an initial and even the main role [BURNETT (48) and SCHERP (47)].

TAKUMA et al. (48) describe that it is difficult to draw a sharp line between normal and affected enamel with the electron microscope. But they still assume that in early caries the prismata and not the interprismatic substance are first affected.

It appeared from the investigation of FRANK and MEYER (49) that microorganisms, can only force their way into the enamel when its structure is previously affected and they present a very positive report about early caries.

2. Dentino-enamel Junction

Already during the creation of the enamel and dentine we see that there is a cooperation of many structures in the boundary region between them. Although the why and wherefore of this cooperation is still not yet clear, numerous facts can still be described about this region.

BARTLESTONE (50) also pointed out the difference that existed in the quantity of radioactive substance taken up in the region of the dentino-enamel junction and in the rest of the dentine.

The interpretation of the irregular course of the dentino-enamel junction in human teeth also varies. Some investigators think that the cause for this lies in the properties of resorption of the recently formed dentine under the influence of the developing enamel. Others think that the irregular course has a functional importance [HEUSER (51), amongst others].

NEDERVEEN et al. (7) studied dentine caries in rat molars, and especially the equally broad extension in to the dentino-enamel junction with various histological colouring methods.

3. Dentine

ARWIL and BLOOM (52) examined the dentine by means of electron microscopy and observed that a perceptible space does not always necessarily have to exist between the processes of the odontoblasts and the wall of the dentine canal. Apart trom this they did not describe many new details. These however, are given by SHROFF et al (53). These authors described that the knowledge about the anatomical structure of the tissues often undergoes obvious changes due to the influence of the electron microscope although it is often very difficult exactly to interprete the newly found pictures. Principally they studied the structure of the protoplasmic processes of the odontoblasts in the dentine and came to the conclusion that the odontoblast process consists of a centre of a labile proteinlike substance, a thin organic shell and a thicker shell made from an acid- and alkali-resistant material that has similarities to myeline in its properties, and finally a thin outermost layer that consists of fine collagenous fibrils. The odontoblast process is then surrounded by a thick, strong, calcified sheath. Fine fibrillary trabeculae connect the outermost shell of the process and the fibrils of the intertubular matrix on the other side. Moreover there is still a fibrillary collagenous shell between the calcified sheath and this matrix. The investigators think that on account of their observations the nomenclature concerning these various layers should be changed. LENTZ (54) finds that the extensions of the odontoblasts completely fill the small dentinal tubules and thus cannot be swollen up in the first stage of caries as is supposed. Bacteria were only observed by him in carious dentine in the outermost layers of the softened dentine. More deeply in the small dentine canals he found calcium crystals and wreckage of the destroyed odontoblast processes that were previously regarded as being bacteria.

D. Summary

Histological knowledge of dental tissue in recent years has changed due especially to the advances in investigation by making use of radioactive isotopes and the electron microscope. It may be said that each stage of development of the dental tissue and the dental tissue already formed should be subjected to an investigation with these new technical facilities. Most of the pictures obtained with the electron microscope cannot however be interpreted with absolute certainty; several observations, amongst others of the odontoblast extensions, indicate that the dental structure evidently in some degree deviates from the ideas that up to the present day were conceived by using the ordinary microscope. As with the ordinary microscope one is equally limited with the electron microscope to the limits of magnifying ability. One also remains temporary checked by the fact that only very thin sections can be made on account of the hard dental tissue when this is previously decalcified This can result in possible changes in structure.

Several investigators attempted to carry out a more systematic investigation by first studying the normal formation of the dental tissue and the structures of the completed tissue and then by studying the pathological events taking place in the tissue.

III. Dental Caries and General Health

A. Introduction

In 1910 WILLIAM HUNTER (55) had already drawn attention to the harmful influences that badly treated dental roots under jacket crowns and bridges have on the general health.

It is especially inflammation arising after caries has commenced in the hard dental tissue that can progress to a granuloma on the root tip and eventually still further progress to cause much damage.

It was ROSENOW (56) in particular who developed the theory that infectious foci of dental origin are the cause for a number of diseases and especially those of the joints.

Although most of the more recent publications were nearly all exclusively based on clinical observations and impressions, numerous suspicious teeth were sacrificed during the next 30 years in the belief that by this means lesions of the kidneys, heart and joints would be cured.

During the last 20 years one has begun to study this question using supplementary diagnostic methods. Thus, in 1951 we find a complete number of the Journal of the American Dental Association devoted to a report about the present-day position of the problem of „focal infection". The 59 subdivisions are summarized in 6 chapters. It is pointed out that a transient bacteraemia occurs following dental extraction and especially when the oral mucosa is inflamed. However it appears that after 10 minutes the bacteria in the circulation are rendered harmless. One has to consider that it is only for a number of known bacteria that this course of events can be demonstrated. The bacteraemia following these extractions cannot be completely rendered harmless under certain conditions and it is then that the authors again point out that one should not underestimate the danger of infected milk teeth with fistulae becoming sources of focal infection [LAUTENBACH (67,58)].

It appears from the whole report that the importance of focal infection in America is regarded with some scepticism since the problems associated with this are not explained satisfactorily from the classical theories, which are that the bacteria or their toxins are transported via the circulation to another part of the body and there excite signs of inflammation.

Thus, although the period of overstressing the importance of focal infection must be dismissed to the past there must still frequently be warned against an unmotivated scepticism which can easily result in reduced vigilence. For this reason KOLMER (5) as well as HEMMELER (60) advocated a reassessment of the problem of focal infection. RUSHTON (61) says that everyone is convinced of the importance of healthy teeth for the general state of health but has abandoned the idea previously believed that focal infection can be held responsible for a number of specific and chronic diseases. This was not because the possibility was doubted that an infectious focus in the mouth can lead to progressive inflammatory lesions [either via the tissues (osteomyelitis), via the surface to the mucosa or via the circulation (such as in subacute bacterial endocarditis)] but that the belief is no longer held that diseases such as arthritis, rheumatism and nephritis in general arise in this way.

B. Some Particular Aspects

In recent years we find occasional reference in the literature to investigations concerning the problems mentioned.

This literature will be discussed below in the chronological order. It reveals how difficult it is to demonstrate a connection between the general state of health and dental caries.

1. Bacteraemia and Cardiac Lesions

As has already been mentioned above bacteria can enter the circulation as a result of the dentists intervention and extractions in particular. In 1956 BEECHEN et al. (62) by means of blood cultures investigated the possibility if this was also the case after amputation of a living dental pulp. All the cultures were negative with the exception of one. However contamination of this one blood sample could not be excluded. In general the microorganisms in the blood are rendered harmless very quickly [JAWETZ (63)]. However there are certain exceptions to this rule. Streptococcus viridans is particularly important. MATTHEWS (64) in 1950 pointed out that these are normally found in the oral cavity. When for one reason or another they enter the blood then they are rapidly rendered harmless unless certain cardic lesions exist, especially those of the valves, in which these bacteria can thrive and thus cause endocarditis lenta.

The microorganisms cannot only cause bacteraemia as a result of extractions. They can also appear apparently spontaneously in the circulation when an infected focus is present in the oral cavity (granuloma and pockets).

2. Provocation Drugs

When one does not regard the mechanism of focal infection any more as a simple metastasizing of bacteria but as an antigen depot, against which antibodies are formed, then a clinical manifestation can result when the antigen and antibodies meet. A certain connection can be demonstrated between joint lesions and root granulomas present at the same time by using various tests (amongst others the BOTTYAN test (65 and 66). In 1954 DRIAK (67) presented a review of the methods to provocate dental foci. He applied weak X-rays. In 1950 HUNEKE (68) described the use of impletol to trace foci in the mouth that could be held responsible for certain morbid symptoms.

3. The Milk Teeth

The milk teeth are affected in a very high percentage of toddlers. Fistulas and abscesses often occur in the mouth. Extraction of the milk teeth causes these fistulas and abscesses rapidly to disappear so that this therapy usually seems to be indicated. However from the point of view of the orthodontist there are disadvantages in extracting the milk teeth too early as these act as natural space retainers. After extraction all manner of undesired displacements take place in the second dentition. It has not yet been established that the abscesses are indeed damaging to the general health and one will thus be inclined to listen to the advice of the orthodontist.

KEYSER (69) supposed that a connection existed between abscesses in the mouth and a poor general state of health. He points out that in order to prevent many unpleasant results early conservative treatment of course is more suitable than early extraction when fistulas have occurred. Conservative treatment of all the toddlers however cannot be put into practice for the time being.

4. Bronchitis

In 1949 VENEKLAAS and MAANEN (70) described a patient of $4\frac{1}{2}$ years old in whom the diagnosis of recurring bronchitis with bronchopneumonia was made. An investigation for allergy in this patient was negative; examination of the tonsils, adenoids and nasal sinuses showed them to be normal.

Extensive caries was found on the 4 molars of the second dentition. The mouth flora appeared to contain haemolytic streptococci. The caries was removed from the teeth and a vaccine of haemolytic streptococci was injected subcutaneously for 5 months. After one month the general condition had already improved. The authors think that there was a relation between the pulmonary lesion and the carious process in the mouth although the evidence is not conclusive.

5. The Eyes

In 1949 McGHEE (71) described the improvements in intraocular lesions after infectious foci in the teeth had been removed. He wondered however if the improvement had been the same when the focus in the mouth had not been treated. According to McGHEE the theory of focal infection relies too much on clinical data and the proof is not objective enough.

6. Systemic Diseases

ROCKOFF et al. (72) also pointed out that lesions in the mouth are found to underly different systemic diseases. He presented a review of this and in particular of processes affecting the buccal mucosa. But one can also find similar lesions in deficiency diseases e. g. vitamine deficiency, amongst others.

7. Diabetes

NICHOLS and SHAW (73) investigated whether there was any connection between diabetes mellitus and the susceptibility to caries by means of tests on caries-sensitive rats. Although it is doubtful if the results in rats can be applied to man, this investigation certainly gives an indication that no direct relation exists between diabetes and caries. ULRICH (74) carried out a clinical investigation in 375 patients with diabetes and came to the conclusion that the frequency of caries in young diabetics is less than in healthy people of the same age. He then discussed the possible causes for this.

C. Summary

The problem of the connection between dental caries and the general health is dependent to a great extent on the bacteriological and immunological state.

After World War II a sceptical attitude has developed as regards the theory of focal infection. But there still remain devoted adherents to this theory who render the patient toothless and tonsilless.

When we read the literature of recent years then it appears that it is regularly attempted to demonstrate a connection between caries and a certain disease or morbid symptoms. We cannot really speak of a great advance of the knowledge concerning this question.

IV. Dental Caries and Hormones

The study of the influence of hormones on dental caries can almost exclusively be carried out in animals. It is certain that the influence of the endocrine glands cannot be neglected; yet it will be clear that practical application is not possible on a large scale or is even hardly possible at all. In any case, experiments on animals made a number of important observations possible, especially on the correlations between the functions of several organs. SHAFER and MUHLER (75), in a survey, discussed the studies made in the endocrinological field. Little is known about the influence of parathyroid glands, adrenal glands and pancreas. The same applies to the pituitary gland. In general, it may be said, however, that since the pituitary gland affects all other endocrine glands, functional disturbances of this gland are bound to have some effect. Much more is known about the interaction between the gonads or sex hormones and dental caries, and also about the effects which the thyroid and salivary glands have on the teeth. Although the latter are not endocrine glands in the strict sense of the word, they should also be discussed in this connection.

BIXLER, MUHLER and SHAFER (76) repeatedly observed that orchiectomy substantially reduces dental caries in male rats. The effect of ovariectomy in female rats was somewhat less constant, both a decrease and an increase in caries being possible. This finding confirmed the work carried out by SHAW (77) in 1950. The same result was found in hamsters [SHAFER and HEIN (78)], so that the findings of KEYES (79), in 1948, were also confirmed again. However, GRANADOS, GLAVIND and DAM (80) could not observe this effect.

It is worth noting that normal male hamsters are more caries susceptible than are female hamsters. In rats, such distinct differences between the sexes are not found.

The effects described above have partly been looked upon as a secondary effect, because the salivary glands, in addition to showing histological differences in male and female animals, exhibit particular alterations following castration. Salivariectomy always brings about an increase in the incidence of caries, as has been observed by many investigators [CHEYNE (81), GILDA and KEYES (82), SCHWARTZ and WEISBERGER (83)]. Yet, castration has also effect in salivariectomized

animals. From this it must be concluded that sex hormones also –
perhaps even for the greater part – affect dental caries directly and not
through the salivary glands only. This opinion is corroborated by the
finding that injections with oestradiol and diaethyl-oestradiol or
testosterone into castrated animals increase the incidence of caries
again up to control values. Methylandrostenediol however, does not
have this effect. It makes no difference whether or not the animals are
previously submitted to salivariectomy, although animals without
salivary glands always develop more caries than do animals which are
normal in this respect.

Yet, an interaction between gonads and salivary glands cannot be
excluded, since BIXLER, MUHLER and SHAFER (84) noticed that the
weight of the testes decreased and that of the uterus increased after
salivariectomy, whereas AFONSKI (85) observed a reduced reproduction
in albino mice. However, the action of the salivary glands is linked
much more closely with that of the thyroid glands. BIXLER, MUHLER
and SHAFER (86) also studied this subject thoroughly. It appeared that
dried thyroid powder reduces dental caries. The same effect is produced
by thyroxine injections. Thyroidectomy or administration of thiouracil,
as well as of radioactive iodine (which causes atrophy of the thyroid
gland) gave a reduced resistance to caries. Futhermore, the salivary
glands also exhibit atrophy after administration of radioactive iodine.
According to RYAN and KIRKWOOD (87), the submaxillary and parotid
glands play a role in the regulation of the blood thyroxine concentration
in that they break down thyroxine while liberating iodine-ions. Consequently, the iodine finds its way into the saliva and can resume its cycle
via the intestinal tract. Thus, the salivary glands concentrate iodine.
Clinically, hypersalivation is frequently observed in cases of hyper-
thyroidism and, conversely, atrophy of the salivary glands is found in
patients with myxoedema. Naturally, it might be expected that radioactive iodine also has a direct injurious effect on the salivary glands.
By administering thyroxine to thyroidectomized rats, it was possible
to reduce the incidence of caries to control values and to normalize
the basal metabolism.

Atrophy of the salivary glands is accompanied by a decreased
amylase activity in the saliva. According to SHAFER, CLARK and
MUHLER (88) the proteolytic activity is also reduced. This effect was
also observed by SREEBNY (89). WILLET, RESNICK and SHAW (90) demonstrated, moreover, that the protease level of the saliva is also determined
genetically and that there need not necessarily be a direct relation to
the susceptibility to dental caries. The atrophy of the salivary glands in

the last-mentioned studies was observed in rats after hypophysectomy and the histological alterations were exactly the same as those found when the activity of the thyroid glands was reduced by the above-mentioned measures.

Whatever the effects of hormones, little is known about the mechanism of the reactions. The observations discussed here show that there is hardly any therapeutical possibility. It should be kept in mind, however, that particular therapeutic measures for other purposes (e.g. sex hormones, thyroxine, etc., and perhaps adrenocortical hormones) may have side effects on the dentition.

V. Observations in Man

A. Introduction

Many theories for the occurence of dental caries are based on observations in population groups. Actually is was found that in primitive people often little or no caries is found. When these primitive people follow a more modern way of life then caries usually developes very quickly. The majority of the investigators suppose that the diet must be the main reason for this difference.

The diet of primitive people varies in many respects from that of modern man. When primitive people change to a modern way of life they usually assume the eating habits of the Western world very quickly. But it must still be emphasized that the diet is only one aspect of the problem. In many other respects the conditions of life also vary in primitive people very much from those of modern man. We will try to give a few examples of these sorts of observations in chronological order. It is impossible to give a complete survey; for this one is referred to the review of the literature by Toverud et al. This was compiled for the National Research Council (91).

One should realise in these observations that what one establishes are only *correlations* and nothing more. It is never proved that the one should be the cause of the other. For this purpose experiments are necessary and where possible with men, otherwise with animals.

B. Tropical Regions

Orr and Gilkes (92) carried out an extensive investigation into the Kikuyu and Masai tribes in Kenya. The former only eat a vegetable diet (maize, sweet potatoes, etc.) and the latter group have a diet consisting entirely of animal products (meat, milk, blood). 13.7 % of the Kikuyu children had caries as against only 1.6 % of the Masai boys and 3.6 % of the Masai girls. It is not easy to indicate a definite cause for this difference. The animal diet of the Masai is undoubtedly better in many respects than the vegetable diet of the Kikuyu However, there can also be other factors apart from the diet that may be of influence. The standard of life of both groups varies in many respects.

FERGUSON (93 and 94) was the first person to investigate the teeth of natives of American Samoa. A very obvious correlation existed between the degree of „civilization" and caries. 1.7 % of carious teeth and molars were found in school children living around the port. This figure dropped to 0.83 % in a school 13 miles from the port and 0.19 % in a „jungle" school. The parents of the children of the school situated near the port all worked for the American Navy, earned high wages and for this reason bought mainly white flour, sugar and sugar products. More inland there was not so much money available and the goods were more expensive on account of the costs of transport. There were no Western articles of food at all in the „jungle" school.

ORANJE, NORISKIN and OSBORN (95) examined different groups of Bantu's, tribes still living according to their original primitive manner and groups consisting of those who worked in the mines and those who sought work in the town. The latter group were able to buy modern Western products from the neighbouring shops with the money that they earned. These products consisted mainly of white flour, sugar and sugar products. In the primitive people 36 % of the adults examined had caries, 56 % of the mineworkers and 68 % of those working in the town.

In 1934 MELLANBY (96) was also struck by the low frequency of caries in different parts of Africa. Caries was found in 16 % of young adults examined in Kenya; 80 % of the Kikuyu merchants present at a market appeared to be free of caries. Young adults and adults were examined at a school in Rhodesia; 50 % of the children had caries as opposed to 5 % of the adults. Vitamines were thought to be a factor influencing these figures: the children were clothed as far as possible where as the adults that were present had not worn clothes during their youth and thus were far more used to being exposed to the sun.

CLOWSON (97) was struck by the extremely good teeth of the nomad Bedouins. The average caries percentage was 1.5 %. This percentage rapidly rose to 18 % in a group of Bedouins who were employed by a Western concern. It was noticeable that many „pits" and deep fissures were found in the teeth of the nomad Bedouins. Usually these lesions quickly become carious. However, in these nomad Bedouins this was not so. This author also attached much value to the diet. Amongst the nomad Bedouins this consisted of cerials, still ground in a primitive manner, much milk, butter and cheese (made from camel milk) and camel meat.

TAYLOR and DAY (98) and DAY and TANDAN (99) reported their findings in India. Very good teeth (1.4 cavities per child) were found in children from the Punjab, who had a shortage of vitamin D and calcium in their diet. Thus vitamin D and calcium could not be of any influence. These authors attached great importance to the cleansing action of the primitive, raw diet. In 26 children in an orphanage in Lahore, who at the same time had a very primitive diet, 2.27 cavities were found per mouth. In more well-to-do children in Lahore 5.7 cavities per mouth were found. This is nothing compared with 21.8 % in Rochester N. Y. (U. S. A.). In the towns in India everybody soon changes to a Western diet which consists mainly of refined flour and sugar and sugar products. These articles of food have a far less cleansing action.

SHOURIE (100, 101) investigated the children in a different sort of orphanage in India (Delhi) where the diet was more Western in character: white bread, sugar and sweets formed an important part of the menu. 17.6 % of the children were free from caries as opposed to 44.5 % of the children from the town and country whose main diet consisted of whole wheat.

The observations of FERGUSON (93, 94) on Samoa were repeated in 1954 by NEUBARTH (102), who found a much higher frequency of caries. One explanation for this observation is that Neubarts's method of caries scoring was not the same as that of Ferguson. Besides this it is also possible that the frequency of caries has indeed risen in the last 20 years. The tendency appeared however to be exactly the same. In the port 73 % of the children had caries, in regions accessible to cars 60 % of the children had caries, in isolated areas this figure was 42 % and on the absolutely isolated Mantua islands this was 22 %.

Co-workers of the New Guinea Nutrition Survey Expedition also found far less caries in Australian New Guinea than in European communities. 31–52 % of the children of 1–12 years old had caries as opposed to 90 % in Sydney. Causes for this amongst others were suggested as being the total lack of soft, sweet articles of food made of refined ingredients. The calcium intake was low so that no definite connection could be established with calcium (103). In this connection we can quote our own figures from Dutch New Guinea [LUYKEN and LUYKEN-KONING (104, 105)]. The number of Papuan children with visible caries varied from 5–14 % in South Dutch New Guinea. The diet here was most primitive consisting of sago with meat and fish, coconuts, root crops and a few vegetables and fruit. It was striking that children of „Malayean" and Chinese parents also showed very much more serious caries. These children whose parents are mainly merchants and teachers ate principally rice, occasionally bread, sugar and sweets. In Hollandia, the capital, 10 % of the Papuan children had caries. These children had already lived several years in the town and could buy Western articles of food in the shops there. These observations are in agreement with those of others. At the same time we cannot say with certainty that the diet must be regard as being the only cause for the differences observed (104, 105).

We found obvious caries in 60 % of school children living on St. Maarten, Saba and St. Eustatius (the northern islands of the Lesser Antilles). These children had almost a Western diet [LUYKEN and LUYKEN-KONING (106)].

C. Polar Regions

Whilst the diet in the tropics is usually poor in protein, that of the Eskimos, who still have a primitive way of life, is very rich in protein and fat and contains practically no carbohydrate. The observations made on these population groups however agree with those of many inhabitants of the tropics.

WAUGH (107, 108 and 109) worked as ship's dentist in the region of the Beringsea and Alaska. He had to treat many Eskimos with extremely bad teeth. When asked the patients almost unanimously explained this as being due to a change to modern diet with much sugar, sweet and soft articles of food. WAUGH thought he could demonstrate an obvious connection between the quantity of carbohydrate in the diet and the condition of the teeth. Very good teeth were found in the far North where the Eskimos still lived according to their old customs. Some of them had never met a white man. Their diet consisted entirely of proteins, fats (products of the animals inhabiting these regions), some roots and berries.

PRICE (110) examined Eskimos and Indians in Alaska. Only 0.09 % of a group of primitive Eskimos had caries. Their diet consisted of sea animals, some roots, grasses and seaweed. In an investigation of another group of Eskimos living in or near the settlement caries was found in 13 % of them. They obtained their articles of food mainly from the governmental stores and governmental boats. White flour and sugar were bought in large quantities. The results were exactly the same in the Indians: 0.16 % of primitive Indians had caries. They existed mainly on the products of hunting. The animals that were shot were eaten entirely. PRICE found that 22 % of the Indians, who, as the Eskimos, obtained their stores from the settlements, had caries.

D. Isolated Mountain Valleys and Isolated Islands in Temperate Regions

PRICE (111) was so struck by the good teeth of primitive groups of people that he took the trouble to investigate similar groups all over the world. Thus he stayed for a short time in Switzerland. Amongst other places he visited Loetschental, which was a completely isolated valley. Only small paths over high passes connected the valley with the outside world. All imported products had to be carried on the backs of the men to the villages. The people lived principally on their own resources. Milk and milk products, cheese and meat formed an important part of the diet. Besides this they baked bread made of rye that was grown locally. The whole grain of rye was used for this bread which was only baked a few times a year so that when eaten it was stonehard. In this region only 0.3 cavities per person were found in children from 1–16 years of age. Similar observations were also made in other places that were also equally isolated. In Wallis (112) a number of places were visited that were several hours walking distance away from a railway or road. 2.3–5.2 % caries was found here. On the other hand in Vissoie, that had been accessible to cars for many years, 20 % of the teeth were affected by caries. All the modern articles of food such as soft, fresh white bread, jams, sugar and sweets, syrup, etc were obtainable. In St. Moritz where the teeth looked visibly more white and shining (as a result of regular cleaning), PRICE (113) found that nearly 30 % of the teeth of the children examined had caries.

PRICE (114) also visited the Hebrides. In general he found the same state of affairs. Many areas were very isolated. Ships could only visit the islands a few times a year on account of the weather. The diet mainly consisted of porridge, oat cakes and fish. Only 1–1½ % of the teeth were carious. This figure rose to 32–16 % for teeth of children living in ports or places with a regular ferry service. Shops selling fresh, white bread, wihte flour, jam, fruit juice, sweets, etc. could also be found in these places.

In his summary PRICE (115) pointed out that the primitive diet of those living in the Swiss valleys and the Hebrides had a high calcium and phosphorus content whilst the modern diet in these regions contained very little calcium and phosphorus. Price wondered if the differences in caries frequency could be explained by this.

As regards modern investigations one should however ask oneself if the difference in the Hebrides cannot be explained by a high fluorine content of the primitive diet. This was also rich in fish and other sea products which in general have a high fluorine content.

The observations of Roos (116) are entirely in agreement with those of PRICE. Roos has investigated the whole of the Rhone valley using amongst other things a transportable X-ray apparatus. Roos came to the conclusion that wherever there were shops, i. e. where the articles can be transported by road or rail, very much caries occurred. Very little caries was found in those regions that during, or only just before the investgation had only been connected with the outside world by foot-paths. The diet in these regions was exactly the same as Price described i. e. rye bread, milk and milk products and meat. Roos thinks that the main cause of caries is white bread.

The observations by Höye (117) in Norway also suggest the same.
In Valle 35 % of the children appeared to be free of caries as opposed to 0.2 % in Oslo. Until recently Valle could only be reached by horse or cart along a primitive country road. The population should be very healthy. There was only a shortage of iodine (no sea products were eaten). Whole meal flour was used to bake bread. Furthermore very much milk as well as meat was included in the diet. Berries formed an important constituent of the diet. Thus emphasis is also laid on whole meal flour and a well-balanced diet.

MATHIS (118) attempted to explain the favourable effect of hard bread eaten in the mountain villages. The flow of saliva is stimulated by this hard bread so that particles of food can easily be washed away from the teeth. Moreover the teeth are cleaned better on account of the intensive movement of the hard particles, tongue and cheek.

The observations made on the isolated islands of Tristan da Cunha are well known. SOGNNAES (119) carried out an extensive investigation as he was struck by the reports of earlier investigators about the good teeth of these islanders. Originally it was thought that the primitive diet consisting of potatoes and fish was responsible for these good teeth. Sognnaes however demonstrated that there were signs of fluorine poisoning to be seen on the teeth. Thus the good teeth on this island must most probably be due to the high fluorine content of the diet that consisted mainly of sea products.

E. Observations in the United States and West Europe

FERGUSON (94) published the results he obtained after examining 4602 recruits in the United States; recruits from Arkansas (an agricultural district) had an average of 3 carious teeth per person, recruits from Connecticut (an industrial area) had an average of 12.5 per person. The diet of the former group consisted of many eggs, milk, butter, fruit and vegetables. It contained several of the nutrients, known in 1935 (vitamin A, C and D, calcium, phosphorus, proteins), in ample quantities. Moreover these people were in the open-air the whole day. The group with a lot of caries lived and worked in the town, was indoors all day and used packed, tinned and ,,pasteurized" articles of food almost exclusively. The data presented here were the two extremes. Speaking generally the recruits from the country had better teeth than those from the town.

SOGNNAES and WHITE (120) carried out an extensive investigation into the standard of life of 14 children with very little caries and 18 children with much caries (4–13 years of age). The children were selected from a clinic that deals regularly with 200–300 children per day. It was with the greatest difficulty that a number of children with little caries was found. It appeared that in 70 % of the children who had no caries their antenatal clinical history could be classified as good whilst this was only so in 28 % of the children from the group with much caries. It is not possible to conclude from this which antenatal factors were of influence on the caries. The authors think that the diet was at fault and this is also in agreement with animal tests, described elsewhere, from which it appears that the diet during the embryonal developing of the teeth can be of great importance. There also existed a similar difference as regards the conditions during the first year of life such as medical control, duration of breast feeding, diet of the mother, use of vitamin preparations, etc. These conditions were considered as being good in 86 % of the children from the group free from caries but this figure was only 28 % from the group with much caries. Taking the dietary history, especially attention was paid to the use of the so-called protecting articles of food such as milk and milk products, fruit, vegetables, eggs, whole meal flour, etc. In 71 % of the children free from caries more than half of the calorie intake was supplied by these protecting articles of food whilst this was only 17 % in children with much caries. 57 % of the children free from caries had vitamin D during the winter as opposed to 17 % of the children with much caries. The use of a). ,,candy", b). sugar and c). taking snacks between meals, such things as cake, crackers, biscuits, etc. were accurately investigated. Extensive use of „candy" was 7 % in the group free from caries and 22 % in the group with much caries. The figures for sugar were 0 and 22 % resp. and for snacks between meals these were 7 and 50 % resp. Thus it appears from this investigation, that unfortunately was only carried out on an small group of children, that the group with much caries ate more sugar and cakes, etc. between meals than the group with little caries. At the same time it appeared that the ante and postnatal conditions for the group with caries were more unfavourable than for the group free from caries. These differences indicate that the children from the caries group were not looked after as good as those in the group with little caries.

For many years Boyd and co-workers (121, 122, 123 and 124) have carried out investigations into a possible connection between diet and dental caries. We select the following from their many publications.

In 1929 and 1933 Boyd, Drain and Nelson (121 and 122) described how it was possible to stop caries in children. These tests were based on observations that children suffering from diabetes who kept well to their diet, had little caries (see p. 16). Caries did not progress any further in 4 children in an orthopaedic department after they had received a diabetic diet. It was also possible to give 5 children at home and a number of children in an orphanage a diet that did not cause the caries to progress any further. The diet has to contain: 500 cc of milk, one egg, cod liver oil, 28 g of butter, 1 orange and 2 or more helpings of vegetables per day. A disadvantage of this investigation is that the number of children is so small that it is very difficult to establish if the caries had really been arrested.

In 1942 Boyd (123 and 124) pointed out that, according to these investigations, sugar has no influence. Boyd made some important conclusions as a result of observations made on children who were suffering from diabetes and therefore were on a diet. 55 children of $12\frac{1}{2}$ years old were controlled for 41 months. It appeared that the average increase in caries was 0.70 decayed, missing or filled (DMF) surfaces. When one omits 3 children who definitely did not keep to their diet from this calculation this figure in 0.42. The increase for non-diabetic children was 2.0. Furthermore it was noticeable that children who had started their diet before their 6th. year had completely healthy teeth. In another group of 111 children who kept to a diabetic diet the average increase over 3 years was 0.47 for the boys and 0.92 for the girls. 18 children of this group did not keep to their diet and had an increase of more than 1.3 DMF per year. According to the investigator there is no single indication that the diabetes itself could have a favourable effect on the dental caries. According to this investigator the reason for this low frequency of caries must be sought for in the large quantities of milk, eggs, meat, vegetable, fruit and cod liver oil that these children received.

In 1955 and 1956 we were able to carry out an investigation in the Netherlands into the feeding habits of Amsterdam school children of 9 years old. Some of these children had much caries and some had no caries [see NEDERVEEN-FENENGA et al (125)]. Some difficulty was experienced in finding children without caries. It was attempted to establish how much of the various articles of food were eaten by means of an interview with the mother and the child. These quantities are mentioned in the table below.

Table 1. *Average intake of a number of important article of food per child per day*

	Boys				Girls			
	Middle class*		Lower class*		Middle class*		Lower class*	
	No caries	caries	No caries	caries	No caries	caries	No caries	caries
No. of children	44	27	61	64	19	37	48	54
Brown and rye bread in % of total bread eaten	40	23	29	14	28	28	22	16
Milk g	500	530	480	520	480	420	410	450
Buttermilk g	31	24	12	8	13	6	11	1
Cheese g	19.5	14.5	15.5	12.0	15.5	15.0	14.0	14.5
No. ice creams/ week	2.7	3.6	3.7	4.5	2.5	3.9	3.9	3,5
Sea fish g	7.0	8.6	8.3	7.8	7.2	13.0	7.6	9.0
Sugar g	35	53	42	49	39	45	39	44
Toffees, cake g	8.2	12.2	10.0	12.5	6.8	8,7	6.3	11.7
Jam, ect. g	15.9	20.0	13.3	20.9	11.6	16.0	11.9	14.8
Choc., sweets biscuits g	25.7	38.5	25.9	36.4	30.5	37.3	27.7	37.0
Chocolate g	8.6	11.0	5.0	8.0	7.0	9.8	6.6	7.1

*) Social class

	Boys				Girls			
	Middle class*)		Lower class*)		Middle class*)		Lower class*)	
	No caries	caries	No caries	caries	No caries	caries	No caries	caries
Liquorice, chewing gum g	1.8	1.9	2.8	3.6	1.5	2.7	3.0	3.1
Tea g	0.70	0.59	0.72	0.95	1.11	1.14	0.77	0.72
Coffee g	0.30	0.37	0.37	0.60	0.48	0.48	0.38	0.62

It appeared that the children with caries ate more sugar, toffees and cake, jam etc., chocolate, sweets and biscuits than those without caries. The differences were rather slight but significant.

Eating sweets and sugar when a baby and a toddler also appeared to make a difference as the following table demonstrates:

Table 2. *Intake of sweets and sugar when a toddler and a baby*

	Boys				Girls			
	Middle class*)		Lower class*)		Middle class*)		Lower class*)	
	No caries	caries	No caries	caries	No caries	caries	No caries	caries
No. of children	44	27	59	63	19	37	44	51
% that as *toddler* ate								
little	16	4	10	—	27	—	16	4
little to average	21	4	15	3	5	11	20	10
average	50	33	62	27	58	46	55	35
average to much	11	44	8	43	5	32	9	33
much sweets and sugar	2	15	5	27	5	11	—	18
% that as *baby* ate								
little	21	4	8	2	32	—	12	8
little to average	21	4	12	5	5	11	26	8
average	45	40	67	52	58	46	55	48
average to much	11	37	8	22	—	32	7	19
much sweets and sugar	2	15	5	19	5	11	—	17

*) Social class

Similarly there was a difference in the consumption of brown breads. Children with little caries ate more brown bread than those with much caries. The difference was significant when all the groups, i. e. regardles of class and sex, were considered together.

Finally it appeared that when children, who as toddlers had eaten many sweets, brown bread could have an influence on their caries. Many more children free from caries occurred in the group using sweets and much brown bread than in the group using sweets and little brown bread. This association did not appear to exist in children who had eaten sweets as toddlers.

F. Observations during Wartime

Observations were carried out in many countries during World War II about the influence of the war on dental caries. The most important of these are those of Toverud (126 and 127) in Norway.

The following was found after observations which had been carried out on 9000 children in the period 1940–1947. In 1940–1941 2 % of the children living in the towns were free from caries. In 1941–1942 this percentage rose to 5 %, in 1942–1943 10 % and in 1944–1945 18 %. In the villages these figures were 9, 12, 16 and 34 %, resp. and in the country 12, 13, 21 and 35 % resp. The data for different places individually are instructive. In Skedsmo 100 % of the children had caries in 1940. In 1944 this dropped to 93 % and in 1945 to 84 %, but in 1946 it rose to 87 %.

It took some time after the war before the high pre-war figures were reached. This appears in another publication of Toverud. An investigation of 2500 to 3700 children per year from the the 6th and 7th class of schools in Oslo revealed that the average number of decayed missing and filled dental surfaces (DMF number) was 9.6 in 1939. In 1940 this was 7.3, in 1942 4.7, in 1944 3.5, in 1945 2.5, in 1946 3.0, in 1947 4.7, in 1948 6.3, in 1949 5.8, in 1950 4.7, in 1951 5.8, in 1952 7.4 and in 1953 7.8.

Toverud considers that the most important cause for the drop in the frequency of caries is the change of diet: butter, margarine and meat were strictly rationed. The use of sugar dropped from 90 g per person per day to 30 g. Sweets („candy") soon became unobtainable. More of the other articles of food were eaten than before the war. All the pregnant women and all children up to a certain age received a large

quantity of milk (750 ml) by means of the rationing system. More potatoes, other root crops and vegetables were eaten. 95 % pure flour, of
high extraction, to which extra calcium carbonate was added, was used
instead of white flour. Toverud considers the following as being the
most important factors that can be held to be responsible in the diet:
the marked drop in the consumption of sugar and sweets, the increase
in the use of root vegetables and flour of high extraction, that have a
better cleansing effect on the teeth. The favourable conditions in the
early post-eruption period increased restistance of the teeth. (The re-
ferent would like to add here that one must also take into account the
increased fluorine uptake due to more fish being eaten.)

Observations in other countries agree to a large extent with those
of Toverud. Sognnaes (128) has summarized these observations. We
would like to mention the following from this summary. Caries was
reduced by 40 % in a group of children in England during the first
World War. (The figures represent the number of children with caries.)
In Norway the reduction was 15 % in the first World War. In post-war
Germany a reduction of 12, 15, 20, 26, 30 and 33 % was observed in the
years 1919, 1920, 1921, 1922, 1923 and 1924, resp. More figures are
available from World War II. In Czechoslovakia the reduction in 1942
compared with 1949 was 17 %. In France the number of children with
caries was reduced by 37 % in 1945 as compared with 1942 and in England by 23 %. In Denmark the reduction was less obvious 7 and 6 % in
different investigations. In Sweden the results were estimated as being
the number of fillings that were necessary for each child. This number
decreased with 20–30 %.

In the Netherlands the results were somewhat different (129). In
1945 1900 investigations were carried out only in the towns and in the
west of the country. It appeared very obvious that as the war proceeded
the eruption of the second dentition took place later and later. In itself
this could be an explanation for an eventual reduction in the frequency
of caries on a given age. This was indeed demonstrated by the age at
which the teeth erupted. The caries actually increased in older people
and also in the milk teeth as the war proceeded.

G. Experiments in Man

On account of their nature these experimentes are seldom carried
out. Mathis (118) briefly mentioned an experiment carried in a Children's
Institute in Berlin where some children received hard rye bread and

others soft white bread. Caries did not increase so much in the group receiving rye bread as in the group receiving white bread. In recent years however two extensive experiments have been carried out in England and Sweden, resp.

The first investigation concerns a number of children's homes (children aged 2–14 years old) where extra sugar was provided [KING et al, (130)]. The usual amount of sugar consumed varied between 350 and 640 g per week. The children were followed up for 1 to 2 years during which time they still received the extra quantity of sugar, that was mainly incorporated into the meals. Briefly the authors conclude that there was no difference in increase in caries between the group with extra sugar and the group that received no extra sugar. The investigators themselves point out a few disadvantages of their investigation. It gives no insight into the effect it might have had on the future health of the teeth nor the effect on eruption; the sugar was not given in such a form that it remained on the teeth for some time (such as is the case when sweets, candies and especially toffees are consumed). The ref. would like to remark here that on studying the figures of the experiment in Liverpool and Sheffield a certain influence can be seen. As far as the second dentition is concerned caries increases almost always more rapidly in the group receiving extra sugar than in the control group. It is true that these differences are only occasionally significant but the fact that a difference has been shown to exist in a series of experiments is worth mentioning.

The so-called Vipeholm investigation in Sweden had a definitely positive result [GUSTAFSSON, (131)]. 436 mentally deficient patients in an institution received extra carbohydrate in various forms over a period of 2–4 years. This included 300 g of sugar, 345 g of extra sweetened bread, 65 g chocolate, 22 caramels, 8 toffees and 24 toffees. In the control group the number of decayed, missing and filled surfaces (DMF) rose from 15.4 to 16.3, in the sugar group from 16.4 to 17.8, in the bread group from 16.7 to 19.2, in the chocolate group from 17.9 to 19.3, in the caramel group from 15.5 to 18.6 in the 8-toffees group from 12.0 to 17.1 and in the 24-toffee group from 15.4 to 20.3. It could be concluded that sugar will only have an effect when it sticks to the surface of the teeth for a long time, such as caramels and toffees. The effect of the other forms of carbohydrate cannot be entirely ignored but it is effective to a much lesser degree. Sugar when dissolved had no effect but this group had received fluorine previously.

H. Summary

When one reviews these ideas from the literature one must first of all again repeat the positive warning given in the introduction. A correlation is often said to exist between change of diet and the frequency of caries. This correlation indicates no direct connection between the two. Apart from the diet there are many other factors that can change and that can have an equal effect on the caries. The connection is more probable however when the correlations are found on several occasions.

After many investigations it can be said that the teeth of primitive people living either in the tropics, the regions of the Pole or in isolated regions are in a good state of health. The teeth deteriorate when a change is made to modern Western way of life. Most authors think that the most important cause for this deterioration is a changed diet.

The following factors are considered as being responsible in the western diet. The large amount of sugar and especially of substances made of sugar that stick to the teeth for some time. The difference between sticking and non-sticking forms of sugar has been revealed in an investigation in an English children's home and in the Vipeholm investigation. The investigation of SOGNNAES and WHITE and our own investigation on children with much and little caries resp. also points to the influence of sugar and sugar products. These suppositions are supported by the data obtained from the two World Wars when the consumption of sugar and sweets actually diminished.

The lack of coarse ingredients which can keep the teeth clean. Both the diets of most people living in the tropics as well as that of inhabitants of isolated mountain vallies are rich in these ingredients. The diabetes diets used in the tests of BOYD and co-workers have these properties to a marked degree. The same is true for the wartime diet. Whole meal flour and various root vegetables formed an important proportion of these diets. The possible influence of brown bread can thus be declared in this way.

Finally it is possible that the diets resulting in much caries are deficient in a number of known or unknown nutrients. The diabetes diets of BOYD et al. are rich in various vitamins. The same can be said for the diet of the rural residents from Arkansas. The wartime diet in Norway was to a certain extent deficient but on the other hand this was secured against by the rationing system that ensured especially that the so-called vulnerable groups received enough vitamins and minerals. Often they even received more of these substances than they were accustomed to before the war. The diet of inhabitants of isolated mountain vallies is not only rich in vitamins and minerals but also in proteins. The same is true for the Masai tribe in Kenya, whose diet consists mainly of animal products and the diet of the Eskimos. This is not true for the majority of the inhabitants of the tropics. Their diet is often deficient in one or more nutrients.

VI. Fluorine

A. Introduction

At the beginning of the century it had been noticed both in South Africa as well as in Central America that many inhabitants of some villages showed an abnormality of the front teeth that was termed mottled enamel. The teeth and molars had many white, calcareous flecks and sometimes had brown discoloration. It was striking that this process was influenced by the place where the people lived when young. On the one hand, one observed that the people who had come to live in such a village after their 6th. year of life had no mottled teeth whilst on the other hand those who had been born in the village where these lesions occurred and who had then moved away to a village where the inhabitants had non-affected teeth still had mottled enamel.

One was dealing here with something that influenced the teeth and molars during their development and especially during the calcification of the enamel. This factor thus had an effect before birth for the milk teeth and after birth for the second dentition.

McKay (132) must have the merit of finding out that there was a connection between the drinking water and the tooth abnormality. About 20 years later both Churchill (133) in Arkansas and Smith (134) in Arizona could prove that fluorine was present in the drinking water of the villages where tooth abnormalities occurred. They were able to do this by means of newer chemical methods for investigation.

In 1942 Hoffman, Schnuck and Furuta (135) found that fluorine intoxication caused degeneration of the ameloblasts when they are calcifying the enamel. The enamel that should be formed by these ameloblasts also showed imperfections that are visible in the mouth after the eruption of the teeth. The effects visible in the mouth, especially those due to an interruption of parts of the enamel, are due to reflection of the exposed dentine through this interrupted enamel.

In chronic fluorine intoxication however it are not only the teeth and molars that are affected but at the same time lesions of the skeleton are observed and they are described as a disease called fluorosis.

During the investigation of Hoffman et al. (135) it was again found that such a quantity of fluorine could be given that just no degeneration of the ameloblasts took place whilst the enamel, already formed, was evidently so composed that a reduction in caries was observed. A large investigation carried out by Dean (136) in 1939 in four suburbs of Chicago demonstrated that there was an obvious difference in vulnerability to caries between children who drank water either with or without fluorine.

After this in 1945 there followed the first tests on a large scale with the intention of establishing the caries-reducing action of fluorine. The water system of Newsbury was fluorized and Kingston was used as a town for comparison (137).

B. Investigations on Special Aspects

It was equally clear that much investigation must be done to understand more closely the aetiology of decaying teeth and at the same time to find out the manner in which the fluorine content in the drinking water could influence the frequency of caries (caries aetiology). The investigations were carried out in 2 directions: 1.) Laboratory investigations. 2.) Clinical investigations.

1. Laboratory Investigations

The investigations of the hard dental tissue can be divided as follows.

a. Solubility and Hardness of the Enamel

An investigation was first of all carried out to demonstrate the difference in the solubility of enamel of teeth that had been either in contact with fluorine or not.

In 1939 VOLKER (138) described a method to measure the solubility of enamel and dentine in vitro. Moreover he demonstrated that it is possible to reduce the solubility of enamel and dentine by previously treating them with sodium fluoride. VOLKER came to the conclusion that the reduced solubility is due to hydroxyl apatite being changed into fluorine apatite. On the basis of his tests he thinks he can point out that covering the teeth and molars of people with a fluorine compound should also give a reduced solubility of the enamel and thus should be able to bring about a reduction of caries, although he did not demonstrate that reduced solubility of the enamel was responsible for this.

In 1951 SUESS and FOSDICK (139) carried out tests in connection with the chemicoparasitic theory of MILLER in 1878 (140) concerning the occurrence of dental caries to demonstrate that fluorine apatite is less soluble in acids than hydroxyl apatite. Miller considers that the aetiology of the caries process must be regarded as a dissolving of the calcium salts of the enamel by acids that are formed by the oral bacteria. Similar tests concerning the reduced solubility of enamel after the action of fluorine were carried out by RAE (141), PHILLIPS and MULLER (142), MANLEY and BIBBY (143), SYRRIST (144), FISCHER et al. (145. 146). Apart from a reduced solubility after the action of fluorine an increase in the hardness of the enamel is also described. In 1948 PHILLIPS and SWARTZEL (147) worked out a method to measure the hardness of the enamel. PERDOK (148) also investigated the hardness of the enamel and in 1947 he could show by means of X-rays that 90 % of the inorganic substance determining the hardness of the teeth and molars consisted of a calcium salt of phosphoric acid. This calcium phosphate does not have the formula $Ca_3(PO_4)_2$ but $Ca_3(PO_4)_3$ and is identical with the phosphate occurring in crystals in the natural state and which is called apatite. Natural apatite often contains fluorine instead of the OH-group and one then also distinguishes fluorine apatite $Ca_3(PO_4)_3F$ and hydroxyl apatite $Ca_3(PO_4)_3OH$. Both of these, according to PERDOK (141) have exactly the same structure when viewed under the ultramicroscope. As regards the ultramicroscopical structure of the inorganic dental material he believes that when fluorine ions come into the neighbourhood of hydroxyl apatite it is possible that the fluorine ion intrudes into the crystal structure resulting in a greater stability. Perdok moreover also pointed out that this occurs in bones that have been buried for hundreds of years under the ground and can be very rich in fluorine, although the ground and the water in the district only contains traces of fluorine. He states that there are as many fluorine ions introduced into the crystal structure as OH-ions are eliminated. In 1957 PERDOK (149) thought it probable that the increased resistence of the enamel is a result of the strengthening of the composition between the organic and inorganic substances that are found in fluoridized enamel. He bases his ideas on the fact that fluorine ions form stronger bonds than OH-ions. On the basis of this PERDOK (149) thinks that the commencement of caries is connected with a breaking through of the macromolecular protein barrier surrounding the hydroxyl apatite crystals.

In 1956 PECKHAM et al. (150) reported, as a result of an investigation, that strong indications existed that the fluorine ions are to be found for the greater part, thus not entirely, in the inorganic component of enamel and dentine.

However, notwithstanding the above one must state that the degree of hardness is not associated with the degree of reduction of caries [SEBELIUS (151) and PHILLIPS and SWARTS (147)].

b. The Plaque on the Teeth and the Enzyme Action

The plaque found on the teeth as well as the bacteria and debris amongst others gave rise to further investigation that was directed especially at determining once again if the various theories about the aetiology of caries were of any value.

Bibby and van KESTEREN (152) in 1940 and Cox and LEVIN in 1942 (153) investigated the action of fluorides on the mouth bacteria in vitro. From this it appeared that a drop in the acid production of the bacteria could be brought about by 0,05 per mill. of fluorine.

According to STRÅLFORS (154) acid fermentation in the plaque could be reduced by a relatively low fluorine concentration. Inhibition of acid formation in the plaque should occur especially when fluorine is imbibed with the drinking water. Local application of fluorine to the enamel will have a less marked action as this can be no constant influence.

The plaque test of STEPHAN (155) reveals that there is no difference between the plaque of teeth treated locally with fluorine and untreated teeth. In 1953 BERGMAN (156) confirmed these findings.

EGGERS LURA (157) thinks that phosphatase plays a role in the aetiology of caries and describes an inhibiting effect of fluorine on phosphatase in the mouth.

In 1955 PRADER (150) pointed out the fact that 8 hours after the different ferments in the mouth have been left free to act (i. e. principally at night) the degree of acidity on the tooth surface reaches a value that is already sufficient to decalcify enamel with a high fluorine content.

Although the further mechanism of action cannot be explained, BRAMSTEDT et al. (159) in 1955 stated that in caries-susceptible people a certain fluorine content of the saliva inhibits the germination processes in the mouth more obviously than the same fluorine content in the saliva of caries-resistent people.

c. Permeability of the Enamel

In 1947 GOTTLIEB (6) regarded the aetiology of caries as being a proteolytic process via organic pathways in the enamel, the so-called enamel lamellae. Therefore he thinks that the reducing action of fluorine must be attributed to blocking of the organic enamel lamellae. SCHULE-RUD (160) in 1950, BERGGREN and HEDSTROM (11) in 1951 investigated the permeability of the enamel. In 1952 ARMSTRONG and SINGER (161) used radioactive substances for their investigation into the permeability of enamel. BERGGREN (32) also did this in 1947 whilst he used tetanus toxin for his later investigations. He stated that the enamel is more permeable when a high concentration of monosaccharide (glucose) is present on the teeth. But furthermore he could find no difference in permeability of the enamel with the tetanus toxin method before and after the application of fluorine.

d. The Taking-up of Fluorine in the Enamel

Many investigations were directed to follow the fluorine ions in the enamel and dentine. In 1956 BRUDEVOLD et al. (162) stated that the highest fluorine concentration occurred in the outermost layer of the enamel ($\pm$ 0,1 mm), whilst the concentration in the layers lying more deeply rapidly decreased. Moreover it appears that already during calcification of the enamel fluorides are deposited in the outermost layers of the enamel and that after eruption these layers take up fluorine from the tissue fluid and that moreover after the eruption fluorides are taken up from the oral fluid into the outermost layers of the enamel.

In 1952 MIJERS et al. (163) distinguish between the result of applying fluorine to completely healthy enamel and to affected enamel or enamel already altered in structure. It appears that fluorine placed on altered enamel can be taken up better than in completely healthy enamel. This statement agrees with the investigation in 1955 by MYERS (164) who stated that after coating the enamel with a fluorine compound, the fluorine was taken up unequally by the surface of the enamel. The places where fluorine is most taken up in the enamel correspond with the white flecks in the enamel. These white flecks are especially visible by direct light. Many investigators suppose that these flecks indicate only poorly calcified enamel. After making sections through the enamel these places can be made easily visible by magnification. MYERS therefore examined these white flecks once again and came to the conclusion that ultramicroscopical spaces are present in the enamel where the white flecks are situated.

e. The Composition of the Fluorine Compounds

Over the course of years one has come to the conclusion that fluorine can be combined with many substances, and for this reason one looks especially for substances that cause more reduction of caries than the compound sodium fluoride.

An investigation into the reduction of the solubility of powdered enamel was carried out by MUHLER and VAN HUYSEN (165) in 1948. In

1945 BIBBY and BUONOCORE (166) found that the solubility of powdered enamel was more markedly reduced when treated with lead fluoride than after being treated with sodium fluoride. This again gives rise to the suggestion of introducing lead fluoride in the treatment of school children. In 1947 GALAGAN and KNUTSON (167) found no obvious effect after applying lead fluoride using the method of KNUTSON. BACKER DIRKS (168) in 1947 and WINCKLER and BACKER DIRKS (169) in 1947 could establish that there was no effect after application of lead fluoride to the teeth and molars of 158 children. In 1949 KNUTSON (170) still thought that all the fluoride salts gave the same result as sodium fluoride except for lead fluoride that only after 6 applications showed any or no reduction. In 1950 KLINKENBERG and BIBBY (171) found a reduction with lead fluoride when this is applied according to the method of BIBBY, i. e. every 3 or 4 months. CHEYNE (172), EAST (173) and STONES (174) used potassium fluoride for further investigation. In 1952 MUHLER (175) investigated tin fluoride. In 1955 HOWELL et al. (176) reported that a clinical investigation for 2 years on children showed that application of tin fluoride brought about a more significant and effective reduction in caries when sodium fluoride was applied. Since then many investigators have been busy with this problem. In 1956 BRUDEVOLD et al. (162) studied the caries-preventing action of tin fluoride and in contrary to that which one could expect from the findings of HOWELL, MUHLER et al. in (177, 170) BRUDEVOLD found that more fluorine was taken up in the enamel from sodium fluoride than from tin fluoride. In 1956 SLACK (179) also regarded the investigation of Howell with some reserve. In 1948 SCHMID (180) combined fluorine with rhodanide.

The influence of the degree of acidity of the fluorine solution was also further investigated. In 1947 PHILLIPS and MUHLER, and MUHLER and VAN HUYSEN (165) in 1948, PALMER (181) in 1951 as well as BIBBY in 1944 (182) and 1947 (183) think that the acid fluorine solution can oppose decalcification of the enamel better than the alkaline solution. In 1951 RICKLESS and BECKS (184) found no reduction with a 2 % sodium fluoride solution when this has a pH of 3,5.

In general it can be said that a combination of certain substances with fluorine can bring about a greater reduction of caries than can be obtained with sodium fluoride but, up to the present day much more investigation has been carried out with sodium fluoride than with any other fluorine compound so that an accurate insight into the great reduction that is here described appears mainly to be based on the results of only a few investigations.

2. Clinical Investigations

a. Diet

When one decides to change over to adding fluorine compounds to large population groups, one will have to take into account that many food products contain fluorine.

A large amount of data are known in the literature concerning the fluorine content of articles of food but QUENTIN (185) again pointed out that one should take into consideration that many of these data are not reliable since diverse factors can influence the fluorine content of animal and vegetable articles of food products. Moreover many values will be influenced by the method of growth and the soil on which they grew. The way in which they are prepared can also be a reason for alterations in the fluorine content. When e. g. potatoes are peeled, more than 75 % of what fluorine value there is, and this is not much in any case, is lost. Tea contains a lot of fluorine and it appears that when prepared in the normal way about 90 % of the fluorine present comes into the extract. QUENTIN (105) calculated that there is about 1 mg of fluorine in one litre of tea.

It appears that drinking water to which the required amount of fluorine for caries-prophylaxis is added loses 10 to 15 % of the fluorine content by boiling. By changing the composition of the water so that it contains sulphates but no carbonates this loss, according to SCHMIDT (186), can be prevented in areas with hard water.

b. Urine Investigation

Much attention is directed to the amount of fluorine excreted in the urine. In 1956 I. ZIPKIN (187) carried out investigations in Grand Rapids and Montgomery county. From these investigations it appeared that adults excrete as much fluorine in the urine after drinking water containing fluorine as is imbibed with the drinking water. However in school children of 5 to 17 years of age it appeared that a period of 3 to 5 years was necessary before this equilibrium was reached. According to Zipkin this difference can be explained by the fact that the skeleton can take up more fluorine during the period of growth. ZIPKIN investigated the inhabitants of Aurora where under normal circumstances the drinking water already contains 1 part per mill. of fluorine. His results show that there was no single indication that fluorine added artificially to the drinking water can lead to accumulation.

Still many investigators pointed out the fact that natural fluoridizing of drinking water cannot be compared entirely with artificial administration so that investigation is required into the unknown factors. Numerous difficulties had to be overcome before one could estimate precisely the fluorine content of urine. In 1958 MULDER (188) was successful in working out a method that could be reproduced in which the fluorine content in 100 ml urine could be estimated exactly to a few micrograms of fluorine.

c. Clinical Procedures

Although the addition of fluoride to the drinking water is in general the best provision for having a mass influence, a central drinking water supply is limited throughout the whole world to large communities. In 1954 HELD (189) pointed out that one cannot reach the entire population by means of fluoridizing the drinking water and in America this was not even 60 % of the population.

If the decision is made to add fluoride compounds then a choice must be made from the following methods depending on the local conditions.

1.) Addition to the drinking water
2.) In tablet form
3.) Addition to kitchen salt
4.) Addition to milk
5.) Addition to sweets
6.) Addition to tooth paste
7.) Local application.

The problems surrounding these various methods have developed in recent years as follows.

1.) The *addition of fluorine to the drinking water* has the great advantage that even during calcification of the non-erupted first and second dentition the fluorine can still have some influence. However each individual varies considerably in his eating and drinking habits so that it becomes necessary to study these problems independently for each country and various population groups. In 1958 the American Medical Association (190) in considering this problem again reported that, according to them, fluoridation of the drinking water is a safe method to combat caries. In recent publications however many differ in their interpretation of the value of fluoridation the drinking water. In 1955 AST et al. (137) described their results after fluoridizing the drinking water in Newburgh for 8 years. Kingston was used as a control. Apart

from clinical observations the results of X-ray examination were analysed at the same time. 756 children aged from 6 to 10 years were concerned in the investigation. It appeared that the DMF rate in the children
from Newburgh was 60 % lower than that for the children from Kingston.
The number of children between 6 and 9 years of age with caries-free
milk teeth was three times as great as in Kingston. Moreover the writers
thought they could state that the approximal surfaces are better pro-
tected by fluorine than the occlusal surfaces. In 1956 HILL et al. (191)
described their results after fluoridizing the drinking water of Evanston
for 8½ years. The investigation concerned children aged 6 to 8 years
old who had experienced the effect of fluoridation both pre- and postnatally. The average reduction is 64 %. It was noticed that the increase
of the number of children with a low lactobacilli content of the saliva
appears to be statistically significant. Similarly those children with high
lactobacilli values showed a decrease in number. In 1956 ARNOLD (192)
described the results from Grand Rapids where fluorine had been added
to the drinking water for 12 years. Both the first and second dentition
of children born after 1945 showed 50 to 60 % less caries.

In 1955 BLACK (193) presented a review of the objections existing in
America to fluoridizing the drinking water and showed how to overcome all these objections. In 1957 HILL (194), after presenting an extensive review of the literature, devoted some time to the opposers of this
scheme i. e. against the introduction of fluoridation. Finally he pointed
out that in 1957 in America 30 million people already drank fluoridized
water and in Canada this figure was 500,000. HELD (109) states that the
question of toxicity of course remains but at the moment already more
than 5000 publications have appeared about this subject. Still the problem that has arisen with the discovery of fluorine and that is not yet
solved is, how long man can imbibe the extremely toxic fluorine without
having damaging results and what doseage can be tolerated one's whole
life without damage. In 1956 KING-TURNER and DAVIES (195) point out
that in Tristan da Cunha, where the drinking water contains 0.15 per
million fluorine some fluorosis is found. However one should take into
consideration the fact that the population eats very much fish [SOGNNAES
(196)].

Since 1952 the drinking water of Kyoto (Japan) was fluoridized to
a concentration of 0.6 per million [MINOGUCHI (197)]. After 2 years the
prophylactic effect was already noticeable in school children from 6 to
9 years of age but in older children the state of affairs remained un-
changed.

In Switzerland where often no central drinking water supply is possible an investigation was set up to study other possibilities. In 1956 REY (198) paid special attention to the fact that people who drank a glass of wine every day often had extremely good teeth. This caused him to investigate the sorts of wine in Wallis (Switzerland) for their fluorine content. He found most divergent percentages; from 0.15 to 5.5 per million and they appeared markedly to vary from year to year. In Germany the following was stated by the Professors CREMER, MUNCH, EICHLER and KNAPPWOST (199) about fluorides in the drinking water: no other measure has appeared able to produce such a favourable effect. Dangers attached to drinking fluoridized water can probably be excluded to a certain great extent when one takes into account the observations in large groups of people who have imbibed naturally occurring fluorine-containing water for generations. A change in eating habits e. g. consumption of carbohydrates and a life without bacteria is impossible so that fluorine supply to water low in fluorine content is the only effective factor to aim at for reducing caries although, fluorine deficiency is not the cause of caries. This point of view agrees with the statements of British, Swiss, Austrian and Swedish experts.

In 1957 MELANDER (200) described the investigation in Norrköping in Sweden and reported 70 % reduction of caries for the first dentition and 50 % reduction for the second dentition. The writer remarks that also in the mouths of children who imbibe water containing fluorine many milk teeth were found to be severely damaged. In 1957 SELLMAN et al. (201) presented a report about an investigation in South Sweden. In this the following results, amongst others, were reported: no difference was found between fluorine and non-fluorine districts as far as the number of erupted teeth in the eruption stage of the second molars was concerned: furthermore the preventive influence of fluorine was likewise revealed in children who had not always lived in the fluorine districts. Thus here a clear influence was observed on the enamel of teeth already erupted.

KEMP (202), BROMEHEAD (203), MAC WHINNI (204), HOUSER and KNOX (205) and WALDBOTT (206) all describe observations in people from districts where the water contains 1 per million or less of fluorine and where still the so-called mottled teeth occur as the first sign of fluorosis. From the above it also appears that the lesions in the teeth arise after the imbibition of very diverging quantities of fluorine. In 1958 STEYN (207) therefore again points out that fluorine is a toxic substance for man which can give rise to toxic signs when imbibed chronicly.

Thus in 1958 the problem existed if in order to reduce the amount of dental caries man must be exposed to possible fluorine intoxication.

This is all the more so since supplying fluorine does not solve the caries problem but is only one aspect of caries prophylaxis.

2.) Action in tablet form. It was already mentioned above that it is only a small part of the world population that can obtain its drinking water from water works. Thus for a large percentage of people other possible means instead of fluoridizing the drinking water must be sought. One of these possibilities is that of eating tablets. Already in 1945 STREAN and BAUDET (208) carried out an investigation into the preventive action of fluoride tablets. However they used tablets containing calcium fluoride which is a fluorine compound that, as later appeared, gives little reduction of caries. Nevertheless it appeared that in the children investigated a great reduction of caries was obtained when vitamines C and D were also incorporated in the tablets.

In 1958 CHRIETZBERG (209) carried out many investigations. He came to the conclusion that the maximal effect of fluoride can be expected during the pre-eruptive stage, i. e. during calcification of the hard dental tissue. If one wishes to influence this stage, then one must remember that tablets should be taken shortly after birth and that this must be continued for many years. The exact time at which calcification of the different teeth occurs is impossible to assess at the moment so that a temporary lapse in taking tablets can coincide exactly with the period in which the calcification occurs.

In this respect the dangers of overdosage must still be pointed out. This danger is not so slight when one realizes that the therapeutic range of fluoride is only small whilst with a doseage of 0.5 per million caries is hardly or not inhibited at all. Thus by the injudicious use of fluoride tablets overdoseage can occur very easily. Experience has taught that the dosage prescribed is often exceeded with vitamines and calcium tablets.

LARSEN (210) in 1948 and STONES et al (174) in 1949 doubt the value of fluoride tablets after carrying out an investigation. In 1955 BIBBY et al. (211) find that the tablet method can be considered to be feasible and investigate if the action of tablets containing fluoride takes place internally (via the metabolism) or externally (directly on the enamel surface). For their investigation they used tablets to be sucked i. e. that could thus be kept in the mouth for a long time and pills that could be swallowed. The result is that the group of children who were given tablets to suck had fewer new areas of caries after one year than the children who were given tablets to swallow. The authors concluded from these results that the administration of sodium fluoride tablets was worthwhile and that the action depended primarily on a direct influence of the fluorine component on the enamel surfaces. In 1954 HELD (109) reported favourable results on giving fluoride tablets to children of $\pm$ 6 years of age. The investigation took 3 years and, as was expected, the first molars showed that they had been influenced by the tablets to a much lesser extent than all the other secondary teeth; the development of the crowns of the first molars was already mainly completed when the tablets were first taken. In 1958 KESSLER (212) reported good results using sodium fluoride tablets given to children of 6 to 10 years of age for 3 years. The reduction of caries of the secondary dentition reached an average of 30 %. The administration of fluoride tablets seems an attractive way of taking fluoride but there are still so many objections or unknown factors to take into consideration that the era for administration to large population groups has not yet arrived.

3.) Addition to salt. In Switzerland iodine has been added to salt for many years and it was obvious to carry out an investigation with salt in which not only iodine but fluoride was also added. In 1956 WESPI (213) investigated the caries reduction in school children in Zurich to see how it was affected by eating this salt. Although this investigation is not yet finished the results seem to be satisfactory. Nearly all the objections that arose with the administration of fluoride tablets with the addition of fluoride to salt can be repeated. Moreover it appears that it is actually only the Swiss who are accustomed to buying more expensive salt because a substance is added to it and it will be very questionable how much the population of other countries will be opposed to this.

4.) Addition to milk. Another possibility to administer fluoride is by adding it to milk resulting in the formation of calcium fluoride. It is assumed that the fluorine cannot be reabsorbed by man from the insoluble calcium fluoride. In 1956 ZIEGLER (214) however showed that the increase of the fluorine excretion in the urine following prolonged imbibition of fluoridized milk indicated that the fluorine can be absorbed. It is an attractive thought that so many children of the present-day regularly have milk to drink at school, but still few tests have been described up till now using fluoridized milk.

5.) The action in sweets. The action in sweets also seems to be an attractive possibility. On further consideration the problem of the exact dosage plays such an important role that even when all the publications appear to be favourable on this subject, one must take a very reserved point of view before introducing mass administration. An investigation into this has already been under way for several years in school children in Germany.

6.) The action in tooth-paste. In recent years numerous publications have appeared confirming experiments concerning the administration of substances to tooth-pastes. Tooth-pastes are used daily and it was especially HILL et al. (215) in 1954 who again pointed out that tooth-pastes can be used very well to add substances to that have to be taken daily. In this way one could have found a method that is cheap for administering substances on a large scale. More and more often one sees publications appearing about this subject.

In 1955 BIBBY et al. (211) reported that sodium fluoride cannot cause a reduction of caries in tooth-pastes but in recent years much investigation has been carried out with tin fluoride that can give some result. In 1957 MUHLER et al. (178) reported the result from regular cleaning of the teeth for 2 years with tin fluoride in students. A significant reduction in the amount of caries was found. They also reported that this reduction is only attained when the tooth-paste contains calcium pyrophosphate as scouring substance. It appeared to them that a combination of tin fluoride with calcium biphosphate had no action.

In 1957 JORDAN and PETERSON (216) reported an investigation with the purpose of providing more data about the practical value of tooth-pastes containing tin fluoride. The investigation was carried out on school children aged 8–11 years old and was spread out over 2 schools. The pupils of one school used a tooth-paste to which 0.4 % tin fluoride was added and the pupils of the second school acted as the control group. For one year the teeth were cleaned once a day after lunch under supervision. After one year a significant reduction of the number of carious surfaces of 35 % was found in children who had used tin fluoride tooth-paste. In 1956 MUHLER (207) again pointed out that the reduction of caries in those who clean their teeth 3 times per day is greater than in those who do it less frequently.

7.) Local application. Since VOLKER (137) in 1939 demonstrated that the solubility of enamel reduces when previously treated with sodium fluoride, many tests have been set up to study further the caries-reducing action of local application of fluorine compounds to the teeth and molars. The result is that it is generally known that fluorine compounds that are locally applied have a caries-reducing action. The investigation of SCHUTZMANNSKY (218), and SYRRIST (219) amongst others, revealed that this reduction varies from 30 to 60 % only if treatment is repeated after 2 years.

The objections to local application are that the application to each child is very time-consuming and that it can only be carried out after the teeth and molars have erupted. In 1955 SCHUTZMANNSKY (218) again pointed out that the time-consuming treatment, i. e. for cleaning and dabbing 4 times, should be calculated as taking at least one hour per child. For this reason the author does not advise this method for mass treatment but only for teeth with a marked tendency for caries. These are however difficult to select beforehand. Since 1955 local application of 2% sodium fluoride has been carried out on school children in Amsterdam. Application (4 times in succession) is done on every child every 2 years. Annually 9000 children aged from 6–7 years old receive their first treatment, which takes place in the schools. In order to find out what influence local application had had the data from the „Medisch Statistisch Bureau van het Gemeentelijk Centraal Bureau voor de Openbare Gezondheidszorg" (Medical Statistical Office of the Central Municipal Office for Public Health) were further analysed. 3040 children were concerned in the investigation. When a comparison was made between the secondary dentition present in all the children then it appeared that already after a very short time (20 months) application of sodium fluoride has a most favourable effect and especially as regards an obvious reduction of the number of teeth affected by caries [NEDERVEEN-FENENGA 1958 (220)].

In 1955 SUNDVALL-HAGLAND (221) presented a detailed report of a clinical investigation using 2 % sodium fluoride on a group of 107 children with an average age of 2.7 years and a control group of the same age. This resulted in a significant reduction of caries in the milk teeth of these toddlers after 3 years. The caries-inhibiting influence was noted especially on teeth which were free from caries at the commencement of the investigation.

In 1958 MUHLER (222) reported an investigation using 10 % tin fluoride of which only one application is necessary in three years. Such a high concentration had not been used up to now in an investigation and the subject is certainly not yet closed.

GALAGAN and VERMILLON (223) set up an investigation using local application on children who had imbibed fluoridized drinking water of optimal concentration their whole life. The writers are continuing their investigation as the result was not very marked after one year.

Table 3. *Results of applying sodium fluoride to 3040 school children in Amsterdam*

DMF per 100		Boys 1st. control	Boys last control	Girls 1st. control	Girls last control
Upper					
	Fluorine appl.	13.2	45.5	21.9	52.7
	Control	16.6	61.4	19.6	66.6
	Fluorine appl.	13.9	44.3	21.7	54.0
	Control	18.1	59.1	20.4	69.2
Lower					
	Fluorine appl.	21.4	50.8	30.8	60.7
	Control	22.2	63.4	28.4	74.3
	Fluorine appl.	18.6	48.0	28.8	57.9
	Control	21.6	62.4	26.8	74.7

C. Summary

When one reviews all the literature concerning the question of fluorine one can, as BLACK (193) in 1955, distinguish various periods:

1. Period of discovery   1906 – 1940
2. Experimental period   1940 – 1954
3. Developmental period   1954 –

The literature review above concerns mainly the developmental period.

In this period however a few facts from the experimental period that have not yet been elucidated are reconsidered. First there is the fact that fluorine in whatever form applied does not solve the aetiology of caries but is only one aspect of caries prophylaxis. Secondly there is the problem still present in 1959 of exposing people to possible fluorine intoxication in order to obtain a reduction of dental caries. As a result of many investigations one can safely state that the addition of fluoride to drinking water can reduce dental decay. The problem concerning the addition of fluoride to drinking water was considered in every country outside America separately. This was usually achieved by fluoridizing the water system of a small town with an investigation into its effect.

The composition of fluorine compounds in recent years has also remained actual while facts especially concerning tin fluoride were published.

The investigation using fluoride tablets has not yet reached the stage that responsibility for administration to large population groups can be taken.

The addition of fluoride to salt, milk and sweets is still in the experimental stage. The action in tooth-paste has more recently become of importance. This is especially so since the discovery that tooth-paste can bring about a reduction of caries when it contains tin fluoride.

The objection to local application is that it is a time-consuming method. Still thousands of children have been treated in this way for several years in Amsterdam.

All the literature poinst out that there are still many insolved problems concerning this subject.

VII. Experimental Dental Caries in Animals

A. Introduction

For many years it has been known that dental caries can also occur in animals and, that those laboratory animals having a dental structure very similar to that of human molars are susceptible to dental caries.

Rats, hamsters and cotton-rats are mostly employed for dental caries experiments. Although monkeys are also very suitable for these experiments, even the smaller types are too expensive to be used on a large scale.

For the experimental methods of investigation it is of special importance that notably in the past few years, several investigators have expressed the opinion that the lesions in these animals are also largely comparable to those seen in human dental pathology [NEDERVEEN-FENENGA et al. (7), SOGNNAES (224); CREMER (225)].

The advantages of animal experiments are obvious and of various natures. For instance, the duration of the experiments, although being short in the absolute sense, is long relatively, in the above-mentioned short-lived animals. In addition, the experimental conditions can be much more rigorous than would be possible in man (children). Just think, for instance, of feeding through a stomach tube, germ-free experiments, administration of substances which may be toxic, parabiosis, etc. Also, to carry out certain measures (both exogenous and endogenous) precisely, it is much easier and often even imperative to use experimental animals. In this connection, genetic factors, developmental influences, feeding methods (both qualitatively and quantitatively) can for instance be considered. Another important advantage is that in animals the initial carious processes can be studied at will. Of course the problem remains whether the lesions in these animals can be compared with human caries in every respect, and secondly, whether the results of animal experiments can be applied to man. So far as the first point is concerned, it has appeared that, a few cases excepted, it is very well possible to draw a comparison. The second point will, of course, always remain a problem. It will always be necessary to work cautiously so as to prevent qualitative and quantitative differences from becoming causes of error in prophylactic measures in man.

B. Carious lesions and evaluation

For the caries evaluation, the initial processes are the most important for a good recognition of the various types of caries attack. Therefore, the small microscopic lesions should be studied rather than already macroscopically visible cavities in the molars of rodents, which after all, are very small. In rats, an additional disadvantage in the study of carious lesions is the absence of an enamel layer on the molar cusps, which means that cavity formation has some special aspects not present in human beings (226). All types of lesions known in man can be found in the animals: fissure lesions, approximal caries, smooth surface attack and cervical caries. Both the absolute and the relative incidences of each of these types vary in the different animal species and also with the diet given (226).

Exact recording and measurement of fissure and approximal caries is only possible in ground sections [Cox and Dixon (227); Shaw, Schweigert et al. (228); van Huysen (229)], or in longitudinal sections of non-decalcified jaw quadrants [Keyes (231, 232); Dalderup and Jansen (230)]. Johansen and Keyes (233) described a number of evaluation methods in detail. In addition, Johansen (234) designed a method of recording the eruption of the elements and the pathology of the periodontium.

C. Cariogenic diets

The diets which are cariogenic for the animals are greatly different and include diets containing natural foodstuffs as well as synthetic diets. In addition to the well known corn and rice diets of Hoppert, Webber and Canniff (235), which are cariogenic, irrespective of whether coarse or finely ground corn or rice are used (236), other corn diets, such as for instance the Steenbock-Black (237) rickets inducing diet [Cox (238); Jansen, Luyken et al. (236)] also proved to be cariogenic. On the other hand the Hoppert-Webber-Canniff whole wheat diet is not cariogenic. A non-cariogenic wheat containing diet was also used in Amsterdam and in these experiments it was even the only diet which, in the usual dry and ground form, was not cariogenic for the albino rats [BONTING (239); DALDERUP and JANSEN (240, 241)]. McCLURE (242) observed a considerable cariogenicity of dried processed cereals. The diet contained in addition to 18 % of glucose, dried rye bread, white bread, rolled oats and corn grits. But also diets containing heat processed whole wheat, dried white bread or shredded wheat biscuits, in addition to cerelose (glucose) or cerelose plus lactose, caused much caries, and especially of the smooth surface type [McCLURE (243, 244)]. The first of these two diets was also tested in Amsterdam later on and its highly cariogenic action was fully confirmed. However, in these experiments fissure lesions presented the highest incidence. The experiments were carried out on rats of different types and strains: McCLURE worked with the HOLTZMANN strain; the Amsterdam experiments were made with rats of the Wistar strain.

CONSTANT, PHILLIPS and ELVEHJEM (245) noted a great difference in cariogenic activity between raw, unprocessed cereals and the corresponding refined products: corn – corn flakes, wheat – wheat flakes, oats – oat flakes. It was also observed that natural diets containing refined products and 30 % of sugar were more cariogenic than a synthetic diet containing 67 % of sugar. This synthetic, so-called highly purified diet, which for approximately 2/3 consists of sugar, is the cariogenic diet which has been studied extensively for a great many years by SOGNNAES and SHAW at the Harvard University and by HALDI and WYNN at the Emory University. A distinct difference in cariogenicity between the two almost completely identical sugar diets used by the workers of these two Universities led to the study of the effect of a large number of quantitative minor dietary constituents [HALDI, WYNN, SHAW and SOGNNAES (246)].

SCHWEIGERT, SHAW et al. (247), ANDERSON, and SMITH et al. (248), and SHAW (249) reported that milk powder also has cariogenic activity in contradistinction to liquid milk.

McCLURE and FOLK (250) observed, in addition, that the manufacturing process of milk powder also plays an extremely important role and that more intense heating increases the cariogenicity. Apparently, however, this effect does not manifest itself under all circumstances, as was reported by McCLURE himself (244) and by JORDAN, FITZGERALD and POOLE (251), and which was confirmed by the Amsterdam studies.

Also on the basis of other results indications have been obtained that the variations in the composition of foodstuffs, caused by local differences resulting from the condition of the soil, may play an important role. This point will be once more referred to later on.

Other investigators also tested the effect of diets which were composed according to the actual food consumption of man. However, these diets were prepared of products which had been dried and subsequently ground. Both the American diet in this form [ZEPPLIN, SMITH, PARSON et al. (252); STEINMANN, HARDINGS and WOODS (253)] and the diet of the Dutch population [DALDERUP and JANSEN (240, 254, 255)], proved to be very cariogenic.

Diets not containing carbohydrates, the so-called high-protein high-fat diets, are not cariogenic for rats [SHAW (256); GUSTAFSON, STELLING, ABRAMSON and BRUNIUS (257)], and also E. D. T. A. (aethylene diamine tetra-acetic acid, also known as complexon or versenate), which otherwise stimulates caries, is ineffective if it is added to a carbohydrate- free diet. The effect of E. D. T. A. is local, no caries being produced if it is administered through a stomach tube [SHAW and GUPTA (20)]. Generally speaking the local influences are extremely important for the development of dental caries. In addition to those just mentioned, there are many other measures in the preparation of food, in the method of feeding and in the treatment of the animals which no doubt demonstrate the great influence of local factors.

This is best evidenced by experiments on germ-free animals, as carried out by ORLAND, BLANY, HARRISON et al. (12) at the Notre Dame University. Cariogenic diets produced no caries in the germ-free animals, whereas the controls showed the usual caries attack.

Very similar are the results reported by STEPHAN, FITZGERALD, McCLURE et al. (13); STEPHAN, HARRIS and FITZGERALD (14) and FITZGERALD (258), who gave the animals various antibiotics, such as penicillin, bacitracin, chloromycetin, aureomycin and streptomycin. Also in these cases, hardly any activity, or none at all of oral bacteria could be present. Inhibition of caries is also observed when a cariogenic diet is administered by means of a stomach tube; this phenomenon was specially studied with the highly purified sugar diets [KITE, SHAW and SOGNNAES (259); HALDI, WYNN, SHAW and SOGNNAES (246)]. This measure prevents contact of the dietary components with the dental elements. This can also be achieved, be it to a less extent, if the diet is liquified. Also in this case fewer particles stick to the teeth and are pressed into the fissures. The result varies from almost complete prevention to a more or less marked inhibition of caries [ANDERSON, SMITH, ELVEHJEM and PHILLIPS (248); SHAW (260), GUSTAFSON, STELLING, ABRAMSON and BRUNIUS (261); KLAPPER and VOLKER (262); DALDERUP and JANSEN (254).]

Restriction of the food intake also has a caries-inhibitory effect

[BIXLER and MUHLER (263); DALDERUP and JANSEN (255)]. However, this effect was difficult to produce with the sugar diet, and was observed only in cases of very considerable limitation of the quantity of food provided [SHAW (260)], viz. up to 40 %, whereas limitation up to 60 % was still without effect. Still other measures can be taken. Thus, it is possible to exclude the masticating function by extracting part of the molars [SOGNNAES (264), SHAW (265); HUNT and HOPPERT (266)]. In this connection, mention may be made also of the experience gained by KAMRIN (267, 268) with parabionts. In these animals – the two parabiotic partners – which were joined together, so that exchange of blood took place – KAMRIN observed that only the partner which was given the food (dextrose) orally, developed caries; the other partner, which was not given food by mouth, did not develop caries.

Of course there are other than local factors that play a role. Thus, HUNT, HOPPERT and ERWIN (269) were able to classify the rats in their laboratory into animals belonging to a caries-resistant and animals belonging to a caries-susceptible strain. In addition, the diet has not only a local but also an endogenous action in that it affects the quality, the development and the maturation of the teeth. Partly, it may have a secondary, local action again by affecting the composition of the saliva, either favourably or adversely. Furthermore, the salivary glands are influenced by the endocrine glands.

A study on the relative importance of the exogenous and endogenous actions of a diet was made in Amsterdam. The offspring of two groups of animals – one on a cariogenic diet and the other on a non-cariogenic diet – were divided into two groups, one being given the cariogenic diet and the other the non-cariogenic diet. Of the four groups of animals obtained in this manner, those from parents on cariogenic diet and fed the cariogenic diet themselves had large cavities in their molars. In the animals fed the cariogenic diet and whose parents had been given the non-cariogenic diet, the incidence of caries was also high, but lower than that in the first group. The two groups fed the non-cariogenic diet presented very little caries; no cavities were seen, only some staining with fuchsine ocurred. However, it was not possible to conclude whether this staining was definitely pathological or perhaps (partly) physiological and had something to do with maturation. The group of animals whose parents were fed the non-cariogenic diet had less fuchsin staining dental tissue than the offspring of parents on the cariogenic diet (270).

It has also appeared that maturation is a process which requires a long time and has not yet finished when the elements erupt. The moment they start their function coincides with the possibility of their being damaged by sticky food particles and by the food and/or its decomposition products retained in the fissures. It will be clear that a supply of essential nutrients is extremely important so as to ensure that the dental structure can remain or can soon become optimal i. e. mature fully [WISLOCKI and SOGNNAES (271); MÉZL (272); DALDERUP (241)].

That it is not only a question of quantitative important nutritional components is obvious from the experiments carried out by HALDI, WYNN, SHAW and SOGNNAES (246) at the Emory University in Georgia and at the Harvard University in Boston. The two almost identical sugar diets used revealed an entirely different cariogenicity. In this connection, mention should also be made of the work of NIZEL and HARRIS (273). These investigators demonstrated that the minor differences in the composition of cereals from different types of soils may be great enough to result in a different cariogenicity for hamsters. Thus, a significant difference in cariogenicity appeared to exist between corn and milk powder from Texas and New England. The experiments were carried out with diets containing 63 % corn and 30 % milk powder.

That especially inorganic components play an important role could be seen by the effect of feeding the ash of a non-cariogenic or almost non-cariogenic food [SOGNNAES and SHAW (274, 275), NIZEL and HARRIS (276)]. BUTTNER, CREMER and HARTUNG (277) carried out experiments with the ash of yeast, and ROZEIK, CREMER and HANNOVER (278) with ash of cocoa beans. McCLURE (244) reported that also milk ash protects against caries (milk powder, however, is cariogenic). The action of ashed food cannot or not exclusively be attributed to its fluorine content, and it is probable that a great many mineral substances are involved. Sea-salt produced no caries-reducing effect when given in 4 to 6 per cent of the diet [JOHANSEN, STRAIN, and BARNARD (279)].

When considering which minerals are important, it is clear that calcium and phosphorus must play a very special role, since the tooth is mainly made up of calcium phosphate. In addition, carbonate groups are present in significant quantities. Furthermore, there is a whole series of elements (trace elements) which are present in small or even minute quantities only, but which are extremely important qualitatively and whose presence may distinctly improve or decrease the quality of the teeth. General data about the biological significance of trace elements have been collected by UNDERWOOD (280). In the following, some details about these elements and their relation to dental caries will be given.

D. Role of Some Special Dietary Components

1. Minerals

a. Calcium and Phosphorus

Calcium and phosphorus can best be discussed together since the tooth consists for the greater part of the mineral apatite - calcium phosphate –, although carbonate, nitrate, magnesium, fluorine and many other minerals are also present in larger or smaller quantities.

Despite the quantitative significance of phosphorus and calcium and many experiments with calcium and phosphorus salts, it has not yet been possible to establish exactly how large the uptake of these two elements should be, nor which ratios of calcium, phosphorus and the other dietary components are the most favourable. The results obtained so far show that the composition of the basal diet also plays a rôle [see also SHAW (281)]. In the past few years it has become clear that the Ca/P ratio is very important. Thus WYNN, HALDI, BENTLEY and LAW (282), noticed a reduction of the caries incidence in rats when the Ca/P ratio was reduced from 2 to 1 and to 0.5. SOBEL and HANOK (283) demonstrated that a very high Ca/P ratio (10.4) in the diet caused higher CO_3/PO_4 ratios in the teeth of cotton rats than a diet with a low Ca/P ratio (0.123), whereas it was known from previous observations that teeth with a high CO_3/PO_4 ratio were more caries susceptible as predicted from differences in chemical properties. A similar effect was observed in hamsters when the quantity of phosphorus in the cariogenic diet of KEYES (284) was doubled, whereas the calcium content remained constant [NIZEL and HARRIS (285)]. MCCLURE (244) observed a fall in the incidence of caries on addition of 1.6 per cent Na_2HPO_4, whereas 1 per cent $CaCO_3$ (calcium carbonate) and 2 per cent $CaHPO_4$ (calcium diphosphate) had no effect. BARNARD and JOHANSEN (286) however, noted a beneficial effect of 2 per cent $CaHPO_4$, but only when the diet tested was little cariogenic. BÜTTNER and MÜHLER (287) studied the effect of addition of calcium pyrophosphate and calcium diphosphate and found no effect. These rats were given a (very) cariogenic corn diet*). No effect of 3 per cent calcium carbonate on the caries susceptiblity of rats was

---

*) It should be kept in mind that the Ca/P ratios are usually calculated as weight ratios, as was also done by the above-mentioned investigators. Consequently, addition of calcium diphosphate and pyrophosphate causes a slight increase in the Ca/P ratio. From a theoretical point of view, however, the ratios can better be expressed as ratios of atoms or ions.

observed in Amsterdam (241, 288); neither when it was added to the HOPPERT, WEBBER and CANNIFF cariogenic diet (235), nor when the amount of 3 per cent calcium carbonate originally present in the rickets inducing Steenbock-Black (237) diet was omitted.

However, CONSTANT, SIEVERT, PHILLIPS and ELVEHJEM (289, 290) observed a favourable effect when 1 per cent calcium carbonate was added to the diet in cotton-rats. 2 per cent mono sodium phosphate had the same beneficial effect, and so had basic salt mixtures. So far as the latter are concerned, those containing calcium had a better effect than those without this metal. Thus an increase in the Ca/P ratio was the more favourable in these cases. A definite conclusion is not yet possible. Probably, the relations with, for instance, trace elements, vitamins, etc. have influence on the effects of certain Ca/P ratios. Therefore, it will be necessary to make detailed analyses of the diets employed, notably with regard to the minerals which will be discussed below.

b. Magnesium

It is remarkable that only little is known about the role of magnesium in the teeth, although quantitatively it plays a rather important part. MITCHELL (290) gives the following formula for the composition of the enamel apatite:

$$[Ca_{9.48}Mg_{0.18}Na_{0.11}] \quad [(PO_4)_{5.67}(CO_3)_{0.45}] \quad (OH)_{1.54}(H_2O)_{0.45}.$$

The magnesium content of dentine apatite is probably somewhat higher and is more similar to that of bone apatite.

CREMER (225) observed differences in magnesium content of the teeth between caries resistant and caries susceptible animals, and writes as follows: „In caries-resistant animals the magnesium content was higher than in those susceptible to caries. A long time afterwards, a study of animals in which an increased resistance to caries had been obtained by administration of yeast, led to the same finding. Since the administration of yeast also implied an increased magnesium supply, it cannot be said with certainty whether the increased magnesium content was the cause of the improved resistance to caries or merely a concomitant phenomenon .. ". McCLURE (292), cited by HEIN (293) however, observed a caries-stimulating effect in rats when magnesium was added to the drinking water in a dose of 500 ppm, whereas WYNN, HALDI, LAW and BENTLEY (294) noted no effect on the cariogenicity of the sugar diet.

PARMA, DANĚK and HANUSOVÀ (295), on the other hand, are of the opinion that the magnesium content of drinking water enhances the action of fluorine. In this way it is possible to obtain an inhibition of caries with less fluorine than is usually employed. These conclusions were the result of studies of the drinking water in a number of towns in Bohemia.

Further investigations will be necessary. However, the quantitative significance of magnesium in the composition of enamel and dentine makes it reasonable to expect that the magnesium uptake must also be considerable.

c. Strontium

Strontium may have a beneficial or an injurious effect, depending on the concentration. A toxic effect in the teeth is, for instance, disturbance in the formation and calcification of the dentine [Irving (296)]. Other toxic effects are due to its strong absorption in the bone tissue. Yet, strontium is also an „essential" trace element, as has been especially demonstrated by Rygh (297). Rygh also observed that strontium deficiency in animals produced a higher incidence of caries than was found in control animals.

Barium seemed to have the opposite effect; it caused decalcification instead of mineralization.

d. Manganese

Wynn, Haldi, Law and Bentley (294) could not succeed in obtaining a caries reducing effect with 50, 150 or 500 p.p.m. of manganese when added to the Harvard highly purified sugar diet.

Dreizen, Niedermeyer, Dreizen and Spies (298) demonstrated that manganese is present in saliva in sufficiently large quantities to stimulate the conversion of carbohydrates into acid degradation products. If chelating substances were mixed with the saliva or added to a bacterial medium, the trace elements were bound and glycolysis decreased. Trace metals other than manganese were also bound by the chelation reaction. However, these metals (copper, cobalt, zinc, lead, cadmium and iron) do not affect glycolysis.

For the rest, it is not clear whether manganese would then have a caries-stimulating or a caries-reducing effect. A comparison may be drawn with fluorine. Also in this case there exist problems concerning the effect on glycolysis. Bramstedt, Kröncke and Naujoks (26) demonstrated recently that the fluorine concentration in saliva such as produced by the fluoridation of the drinking-water stimulates glycolysis. So far, it had always been believed that caries inhibition was produced by suppression of the bacterial activity.

However, KRÜGER (299) reported that manganese sulphate or chloride in doses of 0.05 and 0.15 mg. daily, injected intraperitoneally into young rats from the 5th up to the 17th day of life, did not inhibit caries. The impression was even obtained that it had a caries stimulating effect. The caries in these animals was measured after 20 weeks.

Concluding it must be said that it is not clear whether manganese plays a role after all. More data are certainly necessary.

e. Tin

Tin salts are mostly employed in the form of the stannous fluoride or as potassium fluorostannite for local application to the teeth. The effects of these compounds are greater than that of sodium fluoride solution containing the same amount of fluorine [GISH, HOWELL and MÜHLER (300)]. Furthermore, there are animal experiments in which stannous fluoride was studied as component of food and drinking-water MÜHLER and DAY (301, 302) noticed, that stannous fluoride added to the food or the drinking-water reduced dental caries in rats more than did sodium fluoride. Afterwards, this finding was confirmed by RADIKE and MÜHLER (303) in hamsters; the dose used was 10 mcg. of fluorine per ml. (10 p.p.m.).

Important also is, that from the same stoichiometrical quantities of fluorine less fluorine is bound in the skeleton from the stannous fluoride than from sodium fluoride. In 1957, MÜHLER (304) again demonstrated with extensive experiments – this time with 30 p.p.m. of fluorine – that addition of stannous fluoride and potassium fluorostannite to drinking-water substantially reduces dental caries in rats. However, stannous chloride or stannous gluconate had no effect, and it was observed again that the effect of stannous fluoride was greater than correspondended with the fluorine content. The action of tin is apparently closely linked with the presence of fluorine.

f. Vanadium

In the course of many experiments concerning the effect of trace elements on the entire organism RYGH (305) found that vanadium stimulates mineralization, and that deficiency of vanadium may cause dental caries.

GEYER (306) demonstrated a caries reduction when vanadium as V_2O_5 was added to cariogenic food, or when V_2O_5 was injected subcutaneously. However, HEIN and WISOTZKY (307) could not find a cariesinhibitory effect in hamsters when 10 p.p.m. vanadium (V_2O_5 dissolved in HCl and brought to pH 6.5) was added to the drinking-water. Later on, WINIKER (308) confirmed GEYER's finding. WINIKER used approximately the same quantities of vanadium salts, but as the ammonium meta-vanadate, while higher and lower doses were also tested. Again hamsters were used in these experiments. Inhibition of caries was obtained with approximately 0.035 mg. of vanadium daily, with higher doses the effect increased. But after reaching a maximum. the effect descreased again and changed into a caries-stimulating effect when a dose of 0.20 mg. was administered daily.

At about the same time the effect of vanadium in drinking-water was studied by MÜHLER (304) according to the methods used by HEIN and WISOTZKY (307). The vanadiumpentoxide in doses of 10-, 20-, and 40 μg/cc proved to be very toxic and no caries reduction could be seen. The lowest dose used by HEIN et al. (307) can be calculated to be about 0.15 mg vanadium per day, when the water consumption is estimated at 15 cc daily. Comparison with WINIKER's observations shows that this dose is certainly in the toxic region, since 0.08 mg. daily was already more than is necessary for optimal caries reduction, whereas 0.20 mg. per day had a distinct caries promoting effect. Therefore it is necessary to determine the optimal doses very exactly and it must be kept in mind, that the therapeutic region can be very narrow, just as is the case with fluorine.

Comparison of the results obtained by GEYER (306) and WINIKER (308) made it very probable that the nature of the vanadium compounds also plays a role. WINIKER also mentions the possibility of a toxic action of the caries-inhibitory doses employed. The toxic doses are probably higher than those necessary for reducing caries. Therefore, it is of fundamental importance that vanadium also acts locally on the teeth. A change in the lattice-work of the hydroxyl apatite takes place, with the exchange of phosphorus against vanadium [GEYER (306), RYGH (305), MÜNCH (309) and WINIKER (308)].

Recently KRÜGER (299) reported that also very low doses of vanadium given during a limited time (0.005 and 0.025 mg. per day as the chloride, which is lower than WINIKER's doses), still have a favourable effect. In these experiments the vanadium salt was given intraperitoneally between the 5th and 17th day of life.

g. Molybdenum

A beneficial effect of molybdenum on dental caries was reported by ADLER (310). In two Ungarian towns a great difference in the caries incidence was observed in school-children between 12 and 14 years of age. However, the fluorine content of the drinking-water was low in both communities. Spectrographical analyses revealed that only the molybdenum concentrations differed considerably. The suggestion that the beneficial effect was caused by molybdenum was confirmed by experiments on rats, in which 0.10 p.p.m. of molybdenum was added to the drinking-water. An distinct caries reduction was noticed.

MÜNCH (309) also demonstrated a beneficial effect of molybdenum on dental caries in hamsters. The molybdenum was added to the diet in the form of the ammonium salt, in doses of 0.02 to 0,04 mg. daily. Higher doses (from 0.08m g. upwards) produced slightly toxic effects in the blood picture (leucopenia) and caused liver damage. The incidence of caries in theses groups of animals was lowest when 0.02 or 0.04 mg. molybdenum was given. Favourable effects of molybdenum and of vanadium salts on local application to the teeth were also observed. KRÜGER (299) noticed a caries-reducing effect of 0.007 mg. of molybdenum daily, injected intraperitoneally into rats from the 5th until the 17th day of life. A dose of 0.002 mg. daily, however, was without effect. The molybdenum was administered in the form of the ammonium salt.

It is also important to know that copper mitigates the toxic action of molybdenum, whereas zinc enhances its toxic action. These facts also point again to the particularly great influence which differences in the ratios of the minerals added may have.

h. Selenium

Selenium is probably an essential trace element [SCHWARZ (311)], but apparently, very toxic effects are already produced by low doses, and the teeth are also damaged. Since it mainly occurs in corn and green vegetation, which take it up from the soil, cattle often suffer most (alkali disease). Human beings take up proportionally much less with the food, also because the bran, which contains the greatest amount of selenium, is generally removed from the grain after grinding.

HADJIMARKOS, STORVICK and REMMERT (312), in a study carried out in two groups of children in Oregon, observed a different D.M.F. (decayed, missing, filled) rate, which corresponded to a different selenium concentration in the urine. In subsequent investigations, HADJIMARKOS and BONHORST (313) found more indications that a higher selenium concentration in the urine corresponds with a high D.M.F. rate. SMITH (314) also mentions dental decay as a result of selenium poisoning. Conclusive evidence, however, was difficult to supply.

Even by means of animal experiments it is difficult to provide definite evidence. It is known that the selenium uptake is directly correlated with the selenium excretion in the urine. WHEATCROFT, ENGLISH, and

SLACK (315) administered sodium selenite intraperitoneally to adult animals and observed no significant effect on the dentition. The dose was toxic, though. MÜHLER and SHAFER (316) carried out an investigation in young rats, but found no effect of administration of selenium on the incidence of carious lesions either. The dose employed was 15 to 30 mg. of sodium selenite per kg. of food. However, the growth was somewhat less than half that of the controls, and since it is known that food restriction [also described by ENGLISH (317) as a consequence of selenium poisoning] reduces caries [SHAW (260), DALDERUP and JANSEN (255)] the result of two factors with opposite effects was measured.

Another argument in favour of an untoward effect on the teeth is the fact that selenium suppresses the thyroid activity and may be compared with thiouracil in this respect. It is known that thiouracil diminishes the restistance to caries [MÜHLER, SHAFER, (318); ENGLISH (317)], as does radiothyroidectomie [MÜHLER ed al. (319)].

i. Cadmium

WISOTSKY and HEIN (320) observed a depigmentation of the incisors of hamsters when 0.5 maeq of cadmium was given (in the form of sulphate). Lead (in the form of acetate) in the same quantities did not have this effect. The effect was also produced by a dose of only 0.25 maeq. of cadmium. This dose is approximately 14 p.p.m. However, the depigmentation effect is not pathognomonic of cadmium poisoning; fluorine and strontium poisoning also have this effect, as well as vitamin A or vitamin E deficiency.

No effect on dental caries was observed by GINN and VOLKER (321) of cadmium chloride added to a cariogenic rice diet in a dose of 50 p.p.m. However, when the same quantity of cadmium chloride was given in the drinking-water, it had a caries-stimulating effect. These experiments with cadmium were carried out on rats as did LEICESTER (322) in 1946. In the latter experiments, 20 and 40 p.p.m. of cadmium chloride was given in the drinking-water. The cariogenic diet was the HOPPERT-WEBBER-CANNIFF diet. Although the number of lesions was the same, the cadmium caused a faster progress of the carious processes.

k. Other Minerals

Of the other minerals, nothing or very little is known (as yet). Aluminum does not affect dental caries in rats on a sugar diet (highly purified ration), as reported by WYNN and HALDI (323). KRÜGER (299), in experiments identical to those described concerning experiments with other metals, found no effect of aluminum salts either.

WYNN, HALDI, LAW and BENTLEY (294) neither observed a caries-reducing effect of varying the magnesium concentration, of addition of manganese in a dose of 50, 150 and 500 p.p.m., of variations in the iron content of the food or of a change in the sodium-potassium ratio. With these experiments, the workers of the Harvard and the Emory University hoped to be able to attribute the different cariogenicity of their two very similar sugar diets to a particular factor. In a recent brief communication, it is reported that only exchange of the complete salt mixtures had the desired effect, but not in all tests [HALDI, WYNN and SHAW (324)]. It was also reported that neither pyridoxine nor (American) dried brewer's yeast produced effect. Additionally, it can also be mentioned that aluminum inhibits the development of dental fluorosis in young rats and in monkeys [VENKATARAMAN and KRISHNA-SWANY (325); WADHWANI (326)].

HEIN (293) reported in detail on the influence of minerals as well as of non-metallic elements and cited experiments made by McCLURE (292), in which no distinct effect was seen of ferrous chloride (250 p.p.m.), ferric citrate (250 and 500 p.p.m.) and copper sulphate (250 and 500 p.p.m.). HEIN (327), however, obtained a caries reduction in hamsters with copper sulphate. In this case, the dose was much smaller, viz. 10, 25 or 50 p.p.m. McCLURE (292) noticed a caries-inhibitory effect of silver nitrate (100 p.p.m.), whereas zinc sulphate (250 p.p.m.) and magnesium chloride (500 p.p.m.) stimulated caries. HEIN, QUIGLEY and MARCUSSEN (328) recently observed a significant increase in the caries susceptibility of rats and hamsters when 1 maeq per 1. of platina ions was given in the drinking-water.

The experiments recently reported by KRÜGER (299) with copper nitrate were not conclusive. The doses were 0.005, 0.02, 0.04 and 0.06 mg. daily, so very low. Only in one case a caries-reducing effect was observed with a dose of 0.02 mg. However, in a second experiment with this dose no favourable result was seen. A similar study was made with borium (boric acid). In the first experiments with 0.025 and 0.05 mg. daily, the caries-reducing effect was even greater than that of 0.054 mg. of fluorine. Later on, however, no effect on the caries was seen of 0.0065, 0.013 and 0.095 mg. daily. Similarly as in the already mentioned experiments made by KRÜGER, the minerals were injected daily intraperitoneally between the 5th and 17th day of life. It is also important that a salt mixture of manganese, copper, borium and molybdenum salts did not reduce caries; however, if flourine was also added to the mixture, a caries-reducing effect was produced, but the effect was less great than that caused by the same quantity of fluorine alone.

In the light of the newer ideas stressing the role of chelating agents in the development of carious lesions, the studies of HENDERSHOT and FORSAITH (21) are of particular importance. Several salts of aethylene diamine tetra acetic acid (E.D.T.A., complexon or versenate), a chelating agent, were tested in rats, and it appeared that the disodium (Na^+), magnesium (Mg^{++}) and cobalt (Co^{++}) salts gave caries scores that were 3 to 4 times as high as in the controls. The effect of the calcium (Ca^{++}), manganese (Mn^{++}) iron (Fe^{++}) and copper (Cu^{++}) versenate were only slight; the zinc (Zn^{++}) and nickel (Ni^{++}) salts, however, produced a cariesreduction from $1/4$ up to $1/10$ of that in the control animals. As may be expected, the stability constants of these metal compounds seem to be important as can be seen from the stability of the following complex salts, which are in increasing order: di-Na, Mg, Ca, Mn, Fe, Co, Zn, Ni and Cu versenate.

2. Vitamins

Little is known about the influence of vitamins on dental caries and not many experiments on animals have been made.

Of the B vitamins, only the effect of pyridoxine has been studied in some detail in the past few years.

a. Pyridoxine

RINEHART and GREENBERG (329) observed that vitamin B_6 deficiency may be a contributing factor in the development of carious processes in Rhesus monkeys. However, other diseases were also observed; the monkeys developed atherosclerosis and liver cirrhosis, whereas no disease occurred when vitamin B_6 was administered. STREAN, GILFILLIN and EMERSON (320) were able to confirm the effect of vitamin B_6 on dental caries in a preliminary experiment. Animals receiving vitamin B_6 (1,000 μg/100 g. of food) in their diet, presented a dental caries incidence which was 6 times lower than that of the ,,deficient" rats (average 4.2 % and 26.1 % of destroyed dental tissue, respectively). However, the latter group of animals still received so much pyridoxine that growth was normal (50 μg/100 g. of diet). STEINMAN, HEWES and HARDINGE (331) noticed a caries-reducing effect of pyridoxine when rats were given 16 mg. per kg. in a diet with the composition of the usual American diet.

WYNN, HALDI, LAW and BENTLEY (294) however, observed no effect when pyridoxine HCl was added to the Harvard diet in a dose of 1 mg. or 10 mg. per 100 g. This Harvard diet is a synthetic diet containing 64 % of sugar. The dose of pyridoxine given by STEINMAN et al. (331) was only slightly higher than the lowest dose of WYNN et al. (294). It is possible that the composition of the diet plays a role. The diets used were certainly greatly different.

b. Yeast

A vitamin B source of more complicated composition, the effect of which was studied, is yeast. It appeared that European dried brewer's yeast inhibits caries [BÜTTNER, CREMER and HARTUNG (277); DALDE-RUP and JANSEN (240)]. American brewer's yeast, however, has no effect, as was observed by WYNN, HALDI, LAW and BENTLEY (294) and by BÜTTNER and MÜHLER (332). The difference between European and American yeast might partly be attributed to the higher selenium content of American yeast as was reported by CARTWRIGHT (333). Selenium stimulates caries and possibly counteracts the beneficial effect of other yeast components. The inorganic components are probably the most important, since ROZEIK, CREMER and HANNOVER (278) also observed a caries-inhibitory effect of ashed European brewer's yeast.

c. Ascorbic Acid

Of the other vitamins, ascorbic acid must be mentioned. This vitamin affects not only the gingival tissue but is also essential for the development of dentine. However, the role of ascorbic acid can hardly be studied in rats, hamsters etc., since these animals produce the necessary vitamin C themselves. Dental caries experiments using vitamin C could only be carried out on monkeys.

d. Vitamin D and Vitamin A

Naturally, vitamin D should also be mentioned. From MELLANBY's studies (334) it has been known for a number of years that vitamin D deficiency causes hypoplasia of the enamel. These hypoplastic spots are less caries-resistant and thus a higher incidence of caries may ensue. Of course this effect concerns the period in which the dental enamel is being formed. Vitamin D deficiency later in life causes osteomalacia but no obvious changes in the teeth. Vitamin A deficiency also causes disturbances in the development of the teeth [MELLANBY (335)].

e. Vitamin K

Finally Vitamin K must also be mentioned. HEIN (293) cites studies carried out by HATTON, DODDS, HODGE and FOSDICK (336), in which no distinct effect on the teeth was observed in rats, on addition of 1,000 to 3,000 or 8,000 p.p.m. of synthetic vitamin K to the diet. SHAW (337), also cited by HEIN (293), noted a caries-stimulating effect in cotton rats which received 1,000 p.p.m. of vitamin K in the diet, whereas GRANADOS etal. (338) and ORLAND etal. (339) observed caries reduction in hamsters receiving 280 and 30 p.p.m. in the diet respectively. Chewing-gum containing vitamin K was found to have a caries inhibitory effect in students, while chewing-gum alone also had a beneficial effect.

E. Summary

Concluding this chapter, it can be stressed that animal experiments revealed many aspects of the dental caries problem. The important role of local acting factors is without any doubt. The role of systemic factors often seems to be less great, but it is extremely difficult to estimate this. The rôle of the minerals and vitamins mentioned here for instance, might be local as well as systemic or perhaps both, the saliva being important for turning systemic activity into local.

How difficult all these problems are was clearly demonstrated recently by GUSTAFSON, STELLING, ABRAMSON and BRUNIUS (340). Intermittent feeding with a cariogenic 62 per cent sugar-containing ration and a non-cariogenic 62 per cent wheat flour containing ration did not produce carious lesions. It did not make any difference whether the cariogenic diet was given every other day or on three consecutive days. But if the two diets were mixed so as to supply the average amount of sugar consumed by intermittent feeding – 26 per cent –, and the mixture was given during the whole week carious attack was evident. It was supposed that remineralization during the periods that the non-cariogenic diet was fed, restored initial lesions. It will be clear that this opens new perspectives for the dental caries investigations in man, especially as to the food consumption pattern.

VIII. Conclusions

In recent years the theories on the aetiology of dental caries have been amplified with the ideas of MARTIN, SCHATZ and coworkers. The new ideas explain better a number of facts known and will possibly give more starting points for the study of the formation of (new) dental substance – besides information about the destructive caries processes. Detailed histological and histochemical studies of the dental tissues are necessary. Much is already known, but technical difficulties still leave room for various interpretations of the reactions and pictures observed.

Observations in man concerning general health and dental decay – including focal infections – give no distinct indication for an important influence in one or another direction. On the other hand, from animal experiments there are indications that endocrine disorders can have definite effects.

Data on the influence of nutrition in various countries, or in isolated groups of people under certain circumstances, give much more information on the possibilities of influencing the teeth. However, apart from differences in diet, the influence of other circumstances and other factors are measured at the same time and can often not properly be estimated on their value relative to the end result. Yet, there are strong indications that the consumption of sugar and sticky products containing sugar as well as other refined carbohydrates are harmful to the teeth. Restriction of the contact of such food products with the teeth by whatever means must be regarded as favourable. Lack of coarse fibre can mean lack of cleaning of the teeth. But the fibre containing – non-refined – food products contain moreover more vitamins, more fluorine and more minerals in general.

The rôle and effects of fluorine have already been described and discussed many times. Trace minerals have come more recently into the centre of interest, although it was already known long ago that they must play an important rôle in biology. Much research on this point and on the supply of the minerals to be given in larger amounts has been carried out in animals. As has been described research on fluorine is already beyond the first stages and it is applied on a wide scale. However, many points are left that need further investigation.

It is to be expected that not only the quantitative supply of the factors mentioned is important, but also – and perhaps this is the most important – the ratios of the different factors. Knowledge of the metabolism of the teeth is necessary. The absolute figures have to be considered as well as the relative – relative to general metabolism. Even the need of the oral flora for certain substances could influence the teeth locally. Perhaps knowledge of the energy relations of the various compounds involved – ranging from the smallest initial ,,building stones" to the end products – and especially those necessary to stabilize the tooth substances will help. This more physical-biochemical approach has already been introduced in the form of the chelation theory of carious attack. In reverse order, it could perhaps give information on the conditions for the formation or even restoration of dental tissue.

Still much work has to be done. But on the other hand, dental caries could be inhibited already to a considerable extent when using and applying the knowledge gained. A main problem however is, that the measures to be advised are not at all easily accepted by „civilized" mankind of today.

Literature

1. MILLER, W. D.: cited by TOVERUD, G. in: A Survey of the Literature of Dental Caries (Washington D. C. 1952) and also Dental Cosmos 44, 425 (1902).
2. BÖDECKER, C. F.: Dental Cosmos 71, 586 (1929).
3. GOTTLIEB, B.: Z. Stomatol 19, 129 (1921).
4. PINCUS, P.: Brit. Dental J. 63, 511 (1937).
5. PINCUS, P.: Brit. Med. J. 1949/2, 358.
6. GOTTLIEB, B.: Dental Caries: Its Etiology, Pathology, Clinical aspects and Prophylaxis (Philadelphia 1947).
7. NEDERVEEN-FENENGA, M. and DALDERUP, L. M.: J. Dent. Res. 35, 39 (1956).
8. BARTELSTONE, H. J.: J. Dent. Res. 30, 728 (1951).
9. SOGNNAES, R. F. and SHAW, J. H.: J. Amer. Dent. Assoc. 44, 489 (1952).
10. JANSEN, M. T. and VISSER, J. B.: J. Dent. Res. 29, 622 (1950).
11. BERGGREN, H. and HEDSTRÖM, H.: J. Dent. Res. 30, 161 (1951).
12. ORLAND, F. J. ROY BLANEY, J., WENDELL HARRISON, R., REYNIERS, J. A., TREXLER, P. C., WAGNER, M., GORDON, H. A. and LUCKEY, T. D.: J. Dent. Res. 33, 147 (1954).
13. STEPHAN, R. M., FITZGERALD, R. J., McCLURE, F. J., HARRIS, M. R. and JORDAN, H.: J. Dent. Res. 31, 421 (1952).
14. STEPHAN, R. M., HARRIS, M. R. and FITZGERALD, R. J.: J. Dent. Res. 31, 475 (1952).
15. FITZGERALD, R. J.: Advances in Experimental Caries Research, p. 107 (Washington D. C. 1955).
16. SCHATZ, A. and MARTIN, J. J.: J. Norw. Dent. Assoc. 68, 425 (1957).
17. SCHATZ, A. and MARTIN, J. J.: Ann. Dentistry 17, 1 (1958).
18. SCHATZ, A., KARLSON, K. E., MARTIN, J. J. and SCHATZ, V.: Odont. revy 8, 154 (1957).
19. STEPHAN, R. M. and HARRIS, M. R.: Advances in Experimental Caries Research p. 47 (Washington D. C. 1955).
20. SHAW, J. H., and GUPTA, P.: J. Nutr. 60, 311 (1956).
21. HENDERSHOT, L. C. and FORSAITH, J.: J. Dent. Res. 37, 32 (1958).
22. SCHATZ, A., KARLSON, K. E. and MARTIN, J. J.: Experientia 12, 308 (1956).
23. GELLER, J. H.: J. Dent. Res. 37, 276 (1958).
24. PEPPER, M. B., HUGHSTON, H. H., EARLE, L. and BINKLEY, F.: J. Dent. Res. 37, 623 (1958).
25. EGGERS LURA, H.: ORCA, Proceedings of the IVth Congress, Odont. revy 1957, 169
26. BRAMSTEDT, F.: KRÖNCKE, A., and NAUJOKS, R.: ORCA, Proceedings of the IVth Congress, Odont. revy 1957, 201
27. Survey of the Literature of Dental Caries, National Academy of Science-National Research Council. Publication 225 (Washington DC. 1952).
28. Advances in Experimental Caries Research, Symposion of the American Association for the Advancement of Science 1953, ed. SOGNNAES, R. F. (Baltimore 1955).
29. LAMMERS, Th. and HAFER, H.: Biologie der Zahnkaries (Heidelberg 1956).
30. LEFKOWITZ, W., BÖDECKER, C. F. and MARDFIN, D. F.: J. Dent. Res. 32, 749 (1953).
31. MYERS, H. M.: J. Dent. Res. 34, 217 (1955).
32. BERGGREN, H.: Svensk tandläk. tidskr. 40, 16 (1947).
33. BARTELSTONE, H. J.: New York J. Dent. 20, 320 (1950).
34. WAINWRIGHT, W. W.: J. Dent. Res. 33, 767 (1954).
35. ERICSSON, Y.: Acta odont. Scand. 11, 167 (1954).
36. LOSEE, F. L.: Dent. Radiogr. a. Photogr. 29, 23 (1956).

37. BÖDECKER, C. F.: Dent. Rev. 20, 317 (1906).
38. PANTKE, H.: Stoma 10, 32 (1957).
39. TAKUMA, S.: J. Dent. Res. 34, 152 (1955).
40. MAXIMOW, A. A. and BLOOM, W.: A textbook of Histology (Philadelphia 1952).
41. KLEES, L. and KLEES, K.: Stoma 11, 58 (1958).
42. GUSTAFSON, G.: Acta odont. Scand. 15, 13 (1957).
43. LEBER, T. and ROTTENSTEIN, J. B.: Klin. Zahnheilkunde (München 1860).
44. MILLER, W. D.: The Micro-organisms of the Human Mouth (Philadelphia 1890).
45. BÖDECKER C. F.: J. Dent. Res. 32, 239 (1953).
46. BARTHELD, F. VON: Tijdschr. Tandheelk. 2, 76 (1958).
47. BURNETT, G. W. and SCHERP, H. W.: J. Dent. Res. 32, 46 (1953).
48. TAKUMA, S., KURAHASHI, Y., YOSHIOKA, N. and YAMAGUCHI, A.: Or. Surg. M. P. 9, 328 (1956).
49. FRANK, R. and MEYER, A.: Schweiz. med. Z. 65, 164 (1954).
50. BARTELSTOME, H. J.: Internat. Dent. J. 4, No. 5, 629 (1954).
51. HEUSER, H.: Stoma 9, 3 (1956).
52. ARWIL, T. and BLOOM, G.: Acta odont. Scand. 12, 185 (1955).
53. SHROFF, F. R., WILLIAMSON, K. I., BERTAUD, W. S. and HALL, D. M.: Or. Surg. M. P. 9, 432 (1956).
54. LENZ, H.: Dtsch. Zahn-, Mund-, Kieferhk. 22, 24 (1955).
55. HUNTER, W.: Communication on sepsis and antisepsis (Montreal 1910).
56. ROSENOW, E.: see CORNROE, B. J.; Arthritis and Allied conditions.
57. LAUTENBACH, E.: Schweiz. med. Z. 66, 753 (1956).
58. LAUTENBACH, E.: Dtsch. zahnärztl. Ztg. 12, 980 (1957).
59. KOLMER, J. A.: J. Amer. Dent. Ass. 45, 139 (1952).
60. HEMMELER, G.: Schweiz. med. Z. 65, 908 (1955).
61. RUSHTON, M. A.: Intern. Dent. J. 5, 28 (1954).
62. BEECHEN, I. I., LASTON, D. J. and GABARINO, V. E.: Or. Surg. M. P. 9, 902 (1956).
63. JAWETZ, E.: Or. Surg. M. P. 8, 1063 (1955).
64. MATTHEW, H.: Brit. Dent. J. 88, 88 (1950).
65. BOTTYAN, I.: Dtsch. Zahn-, Mund-, Kieferhk. 15, 127 (1951).
66. BOTTYAN, I.: Dtsch. zahnärztl. Ztg. 13, 442 (1958).
67. DRIAK, F.: Intern. Dent. J. 4, 838 (1954).
68. HUNEKE, F.: Dtsch. zahnärztl. Ztg. 5, 1269 (1950).
69. KEYSER, E.: Dtsch. zahnärztl. Ztg. 6, 949 (1951).
70. VEENEKLAAS, G. M. H. and MAANEN, H. J.: Mschr. Kindergeneesk. 17, 74 (1949).
71. MCGHEE, M. W.: West-Virginia Dent. J. April (1949).
72. ROCKOFF, H. S., ROCKOFF, S. C. and SACKLER, A. M.: Or. Surg. M. P. 8, 246 (1955).
73. NICHOLS, M. S. and SHAW, J. H.: J. Dent. Res. 36, 68 (1957).
74. ULRICH, K. H.: Dtsch. zahnärztl. Ztg. 13, 62 (1958).
75. SHAFER, W. G. and MÜHLER, J. C.: in: Advances in Experimental Caries Research p. 137 (Washington 1955).
76. BIXLER, D., MÜHLER, J. C. and SHAFER, W. G.: J. Dent. Res. 36, 571 (1957).
77. SHAW, J. H.: J. Dent. Res. 29, 798 (1950).
78. SHAFER, W. G. and HEIN, J. W.: J. Dent. Res. 29, 666 (1950).
79. KEYES, P. H.: New York Dent. J. 18, 172 (1948).
80. GRANADOS, H., GLAVIND, J. and DAM, H.: Brit. Dent. J. 89, 67 (1950).
81. CHEYNE, V. D.: Proc. Soc. Exper. Biol. Med. 42, 587 (1939).
82. GILDA, J. E. and KEYES, P. H.: Proc. Soc. Exper. Biol. Med. 66, 28 (1947).

83. SCHWARTZ, A. and WEISBERGER, D.: in: Advances in Experimental Caries Research p. 125 (Washington 1955).

84. BIXLER, D., MÜHLER, J. C. and SHAFER, W. G.: J. Dent. Res. 33, 648 (1954).

85. AFONSKI, D.: J. Dent. Res. 37, 965 (1958).

86. BIXLER, D., MÜHLER, J. C. and SHAFER, W. G.: J. Dent. Res. 36, 709 (1957).

87. RYAN, E. J. and KIRKWOOD, S.: Science 121, 175 (1955).

88. SHAFER, W. G., CLARK, W. G. and MÜHLER, J. C.: cited by BIXLER, MUHLER and SHAFER J. Dent. Res. 36, 571 (1957).

89. SREEBNY, L. M.: J. Dent. Res. 32, 686 (1953).

90. WILLET, N. P., RESNICK, J. B. and SHAW, J. H.: J. Dent. Res. 37, 930 (1958).

91. TOVERUD, G., FINN, S. B., COX, C. J., BÖDECKER, C. F. and SHAW, J. H.: Survey of the Literature of Dental Caries (Washington 1952).

92. ORR, J. B. and GILKS, K. L.: Med. Res. Council. Spec. Rep. Ser. 155 (1931).

93. FERGUSON, R. A.: J. Amer. Dent. Assoc. 21, 534 (1934).

94. FERGUSON, R. A.: J. Amer. Dent. Assoc. 22, 392 (1935).

95. ORANJE, P., NORISKIN, J. N. and OSBORN, T. W. B.: S. African J. Med. Sci. 1, 57 (1935).

96. MELLANBY, M.: Med. Res. Council. Spec. Rep. Ser. 191, 160 (1934).

97. CLOWSON, M. D.: Dent. Mag. Oral Topics 53, 117 and 219 (1936).

98. TAYLOR, G. F. and DAY, C. D. M.: Brit. Med. J. 1, 919 (1939)

99. DAY, C. D. M. and TANDAN, G. C.: Brit. Dent. J. 49, 381 (1940).

100. SHOURIE, K. H.: Ind. J. Med. Res. 29, 709 (1941).

101. SHOURIE, K. H.: Ind. J. Med. Res. 30, 561 (1942).

102. NEUBARTH, R. G.: South Pacific Comm. Tech. Paper 64 (1954).

103. Report of the New-Guinea Nutrition Survey Expedition 1947, carried out for the Dept. External Territories, Australia (Sydney 1947).

104. LUYKEN, R. and LUYKEN-KONING, F. W. M.: Doc. med. geogr. trop. Med. 8, 45 (1956).

105. LUYKEN, R. and LUYKEN-KONING, F. W. M.: Doc. med. geogr. trop. Ned. 7, 315 (1955).

106. LUYKEN, R. and LUYKEN-KONING, F. W. M.: Trop. Geogr. Med. 11, 103, (1959).

107. WAUGH, L. M.: J. Dent. Res. 11, 450 (1931), 10, 387 (1930).

108. WAUGH, L. M.: J. Dent. Res. 8, 428 (1928).

109. WAUGH, L. M.: J. Dent. Res. 15, 317 (1935-1936).

110. PRICE, W. A.: J. Amer. Dent. Assoc. 23, 417 (1936).

111. PRICE, W. A.: Dent. Digest 39, 94 (1933).

112. PRICE, W. A.: Dent. Digest 39, 147 (1933).

113. PRICE, W. A.: Dent. Digest 39, 203 1933).

114. PRICE, W. A.: Dent. Digest 39, 225 (1933).

115. PRICE, W. A.: Dent. Digest 39, 266 (1933).

116. ROOS, A.: Schweiz. Mschr. Zahnheilk. 47, 329 (1937).

117. HÖYE, G. M.: Brit. Dent. J. 64, 496 (1938).

118. MATHIS, H.: Z. Stomatol. 12, 699 (1938).

119. SOGNNAES, R. F.: J. Dent. Res. 18, 243 (1939).

120. SOGNNAES, R. F. and WHITE, R. L.: Amer. J. Dis. Children 60, 283 (1940).

121. BOYD, J. D., DRAIN, C. L. and NELSON, M. V.: Amer. J. Dis. Children 38, 721 (1929).

122. BOYD, J. D., DRAIN, C. L. and STEARNS, G.: Proc. Soc. Exper. Biol. Med. 36, 645 (1933).

123. BOYD, J. D.: Amer. J. Dis. Children 66, 349 (1943).
124. BOYD, J. D.: J. Amer. Dent. Assoc. 30, 670 (1943).
125. NEDERVEEN-FENENGA, M., SCHOUSTRA, A. and LUYKEN, R.: Voeding 20, 263 (1959).
126. TOVERUD, G.: J. Amer. Dent. Assoc. 39, 127 (1949).
127. TOVERUD, G.: Millbank Mem. Fund. Quart. 35, 372 (1957).
128. SOGNNAES, R. F.: Amer. J. Dis. Children 75, 792 (1948).
129. Commissie tot onderzoek van de voedings- en gezondheidstoestand der Nederlandse Bevolking, de zgn Polscommissie der Voedingsraad: Voeding 19, 313 (1958).
130. KING, J. D., MELLANBY, M., STONES, H. H. and GREEN, H. N.: Med. Res. Council, Spec. Rep. Ser. 288 (1955).
131. GUSTAFSSON, B. E., QUENSEL, C. E., SWENANDER LANKE, L., LUNDQVIST, C., GRAHNÉN, H. and BONOW, B. E.: Acta odontol. Scand. 11, 232 (1954).
132. MCKAY, F. S.: Panama Pac. dent. Congr. 1, 25 (1915).
133. CHURCHILL, H. V.: Ind. Eng. Chem. 23, 996 (1931).
134. SMITH, M. C., LANTZ, E. M. and SMITH, H. V.: Science 74, 244 (1931).
135. HOFFMANN, M. M., SCHUCK, C. and FURUTA, W. J.: J. Dent. Res. 21, 157 (1942).
136. DEAN, H. T.: Publ. Health Rep. 54, 862 (1939).
137. AST, D. B., BUSHEL, A., WACHS, B. and CHASE, H.: J. Amer. Dent. Assoc. 50, 680 (1955); see also Amer. J. Publ. Health 40, June 1950, and HILLEHOE H. E., J. Amer. Dent. Assoc. 52, 291 (1956).
138. VOLKER, J. F.: Proc. Soc. Exper. Biol. 42, 725 (1939).
139. SUESS, Ph. D. and FOSDICK, L. S.: J. Dent. Res. 30, 177 (1951).
140. MILLER, W. D.: Die Mikroorganismen der Mundhöhle (Leipzig 1889).
141. RAE, J. J.: J. Dent. Res. 24, 235 (1945).
142. PHILLIPS, R. W. and MUHLER, J. C.: J. Dent. Res. 26, 109 (1947).
143. MANLY, R. S. and BIBBY, B. G.: J. Dent. Res. 28, 160 (1949).
144. SYRRIST, A.: Odont. Tidskr. 57, 447 (1949).
145. FISCHER, R. B. and MÜHLER, J. C. J. Dent. Res. 31, 751 (1952).
146. FISCHER, R. B., ELSHEIMER, H. N. and MÜHLER, J. C.: J. Dent. Res. 33, 538 (1954).
147. PHILLIPS, R. W. and SWARTZ, M. L.: J. Amer. Assoc. 37, 1 (1948).
148. PERDOK, W. G.: Tijdschr. Tandheelk. 54, 79 (1947).
149. PERDOK, W. G.: Belg. Tijdschr. Stomatol. 54, 277 (1957).
150. PECKHAM, S. C., LEOPOLD, R. S. and HESS, W. C.: J. Dent. Res. 35, 205 (1956).
151. SEBELIUS, C.: J. Tenn. Med. Ass. 42, 16 (1949).
152. BIBBY, B. G. and VAN KESTEREN, M.: J. Dent. Res. 19, 391 (1940).
153. COX, G. J. and LEVIN, M. M.: Publ. No. 19, Washington. Am. Ass. Adv. Sci. (Washington 1942).
154. STRÅLFORS, A.: Odont. Tidsk. 58, 153 (1950).
155. STEPHAN, R. M.: J. Dent. Res. 23, 257 (1944).
156. BERGMAN, G.: Acta odont. Scand. 10, 11 (1952).
157. EGGERS LURA, H.: Zahnärztliche Welt 5, 269 (1950).
158. PRADER, F.: Dtsch. zahnärztl. Ztg. 10, 308 (1955).
159. BRAMSTEDT, F., KRÖNCKE, A. und NAUJOKS, R.: Dtsch. zahnärztl. Ztg. 10, 311 (1955).
160. SCHULERUD, A.: Norske Tannlaegef. Tidskr. 60, 249 (1950).
161. ARMSTRONG, W. D. and SINGER, L.: J. Dent. Res. 31, 493 (1952).
162. BRUDEVOLD, F., STEADMAN, L. T., GARDNER, D. E., ROWLEY, J. and LITTLE, M. F.: J. Amer. Dent. Assoc. 53, 159 (1956).

163. MYERS, H. M., HAMILTON, J. G., and BECKS, H.: J. Dent. Res. 31, 743 (1952).
164. MYERS, H. M., J. Dent. Res. 34, 38 (1955).
165. MÜHLER, J. C., HUYSEN, G. V.: J. Dent. Res. 1, 10 (1948).
166. BIBBY, B. G. and BUONACORE, M. G.: J. Dent. Res. 24, 103 (1945).
167. GALAGAN, D. J. and KNUTSON, J. W.: Publ. Health Report 62, 1477 (1947).
168. BACKER DIRKS, O.: Communication 1947; Tijdschr. Tandh. 55, 130 (1948).
169. WINKLER, K. G. and BACKER DIRKS, O.: Tijdschr. Tandh. 55, 219 (1948).
170. KNUTSON, J. W.: J. Amer. Ass. 39, 438 (1949).
171. KLINKENBERG, E. and BIBBY, B. G.: J. Dent. Res. 29, 4 (1950).
172. CHEYNE, V. D.: J. Amer. Dent. Ass. 29, 804 (1942).
173. EAST, B. R., ZISKIN, D. E., STROWE, L. R., KARSHAN, M. and RICHARDSON, E. P.: J. Dent. Res. 24, 267 (1945).
174. STONES, H. H., LAWTON, F. E., BRANSBY, E. R. and HARTLEY, H. O.: Brit. Dent. J. 86, 263 (1945).
175. MÜHLER, J. G., DAY, H. G. and NEBERGALL, W. H.: J. Dent. Res. 31, 756 (1952).
176. HOWELL, C. L., GISH, C. W., SMILEY, R. D., and MUHLER, J. C.: J. Amer. Dent. Ass. 50, 14 (1955).
177. HOWELL, C. L., MÜHLER, J. C. and GISH, C. W.: J. Dent. Res. 36, 780 (1957).
178. MÜHLER, J. C.: J. Amer. Dent. Ass. 54, 352 (1957).
179. SLACK, G. L.: Brit. Dent. J. 101, 7 (1956).
180. SCHMID, H.: Schweiz. Mschr. Zahnheilk. 58, 652 (1948).
181. PALMER, H. B.: J. Dent. Res. 30, 363 (1951).
182. BIBBY, B. G.: J. Dent. Res. 23, 202 (1944).
183. BIBBY, B. G.: J. Amer. Dent. Ass. 34, 26 (1947).

184. RICKLES, N. H. and BECKS, H.: J. Dent. Res. 30, 757 (1951).
185. QUENTIN, K. E.: Odont. revy 8, 178 (1957).
186. SCHMIDT, H. J.: Dtsch. zahnärztl. Ztg. 9 (1954).
187. ZIPKIN, I., LIKINS, R. C., McCLURE, F. J. and STEERE, A. C.: Publ. Health Report 71, 767 (1956).
188. MULDER, G. J.: Thesis (Utrecht 1958).
189. HELD, A. J. and PIRQUET, F.: Stoma 7, 213 (1954).
190. American Medical Association; J. Amer. Med. Ass. 56 (1958).
191. HILL, I. N., BLANEY, J. R. and WOLF, W.: J. Amer. Dent. Ass. 53, 327 (1956).
192. ARNOLD, F. A.: Publ. Health Rep. 71, 652 (1956).
193. BLACK, A. P.: J. Amer. Dent. Ass. 50, 655 (1955).
194. HILL, I. N.: J. Amer. Dent. Ass. 54, 454 (1957).
195. KING-TURNER, J. D. and DAVIES, A.: Brit. Dent. J. 101, 262 (1956).
196. SOGNNAES, R. F.: Brit. Dent. J. 70, 433 (1941).
197. MINOGUCHI, G.: Stoma 7, 1 (1954).
198. REY, Ch.: Schweiz. Mschr. Zahnheilk. 66, 1039 (1956).
199. CREMER, H. D., MÜNCH, J., KNAPPWOST, A. and EICHLER, H.: Resolutions, ORCA (1957).
200. MELANDER, A.: Odont. revy 8, 474 (1957).
201. SELLMANN, S., SYRRIST, A. and GUSTAFSON, G.: Odontol. Tidskr. 65, 61 (1957).
202. KEMP, P.: Lancet 6204, 93 (1942).
203. BROMEHEAD, G.: Lancet 1943, 490.
204. MACWHINNIE, E.: Reprint from Memo, U.S.A. (July 1953).
205. HOUSER, A. and KNOX, S.: J. Ohio Dent. Soc. 13, 171 (1939) and Publ. Amer. Soc. Adv. Sci. (Washington 1954).
206. WALDBOTT, S.: Acta med. Scand. 46, 157 (1956).
207. STEYN, D. G.: 31st meeting of the

National Nutrition Council at Cape Town, Febr. (1958).
208. STREAN, L. P. and BEAUDET, J. P.: N. Y. State J. Med. **45**, 2183 (1945).
209. CHRIETZBERG, J. E. and LEWIS, F. D.: J. Amer. Dent. Ass. **56**, 192 (1958).
210. LARSEN, N. P.: J. Amer. Med. Ass. **137**, 832 (1948).
211. BIBBY, B. G., WILKINS, E. and WITTOL, E.: Oral Surg. **8**, 213 (1955).
212. KESSLER, W. and SOLTH, K.: Stoma **11**, 14 (1958).
213. WESPI, H. J.: Zahnärztl. Praxis **7**, 1 (1956).
214. ZIEGLER, E.: Schweiz. Mschr. Zahnheilk. **69**, 111 (1956).
215. HILL, TH. J., ZANDER, H. A., KESEL, R. G., HEIN, J. W., FOSDICK, L. S. and KNIESNER, H. A.: J. Amer. Dent. Ass. **48**, 1 (1954).
216. JORDAN, W. A. and PETERSON, J. K.: J. Amer. Dent. Ass. **54**, 589 (1957).
217. MÜHLER, J. C., RADIKE, A. W., NEBERGALL, W. H. and DAY, H. G.: J. Dent. Res. **35**, 49 (1956).
218. SCHÜTZMANNSKY, G.: Dtsch. Zahn-, Mund-, Kieferhk. **22**, 166 (1955).
219. SYRRIST, A.: Odont. revy **7**, 386 (1956).
220. NEDERVEEN-FENENGA, M.: Tijds. Tandh. **65**, 609 (1958).
221. SUNDVALL-HAGLAND, I.: Acta odont. Scand. **13**, suppl. 15 (1955).
222. MÜHLER, J. C.: J. Dent. Res. **37**, 415 (1958).
223. GALAGAN, D. J. and VERMILLION, J. R.: Publ. Health Rep. **70**, 1114 (1955).
224. SOGNNAES, R. F.: — New. Engl. J. Med. **256**, 1226 (1957).
225. CREMER, H. D.: — Proceedings of the 4th Congress, ORCA, Odont. revy p. 71 (1957).
226. DALDERUP, L. M.: Z. Prophyl. Med. **3**, März (1957).
227. COX, G. J. and DIXON, S. F.: J. Dent. Res. **18**, 153 (1939).
228. SHAW, J. H., SCHWEIGERT, B. S.,
McINTYRE, J. M., ELVEHJEM, C. A. and PHILLIPS, P. H.: J. Nutr. **28**, 333 (1944).
229. HUYSEN, G. van: J. Dent. Res. **29**, 809 (1950).
230. DALDERUP, L. M. and JANSEN, B. C. P.: Int. Rev. Vit. Res. **26**, 235 (1955).
231. KEYES, P. H.: J. Dent. Res. **37**, 1077 (1958).
232. KEYES, P. H.: J. Dent. Res. **37**, 1088 (1958).
233. JOHANSEN, E. and KEYES, P. H.: Advances in Experimental Caries p. 1, Adv. Sci. (Washington 1955).
234. JOHANSEN, E.: J. Dent. Res. **32**, 578 (1953)
235. HOPPERT, C. A., WEBBER, P. A. and CANNIFF, T. L.: J. Dent. Res. **12**, 161 (1932)
236. STEENBOCK, H. and BLACK, A., J. Biol. Chem. **64**, 263, 1925.
237. JANSEN, B. C. P., LUYKEN, R., DALDERUP, L. M., NEDERVEEN-FENENGA, M., BOONSTRA, J. P. and WÖSTMANN, B. S. J.: Tijds. Tandh. **58**, 200 (1951).
238. COX, G. J.: Survey of the Literature of Dental Caries. (Washington 1952).
239. BONTING, S. L.: Thesis (Amsterdam 1952).
240. DALDERUP, L. M. and JANSEN, B. C. P.: Int. Rev. Vit. Res. **26**, 209 (1955).
241. DALDERUP, L. M.: Thesis (Amsterdam 1959).
242. McCLURE, F. J.: Science **116**, 229 (1952).
243. McCLURE, F. J.: Dietary factors in experimental rat caries. Amer. Ass. Adv. Sci. p. 107 (Washington 1955).
244. McCLURE, F. J.: J. Nutr. **65**, 619 (1958).
245. CONSTANT, M. A., PHILLIPS, P. H. and ELVEHJEM, C. A.: J. Nutr. **46**, 271 (1952).
246. HALDI, J., WYNN, W., SHAW, J. H. and SOGNNAES, R. F.: J. Nutr. **50**, 267 (1953).
247. SCHWEIGERT, B. S., SHAW, J. H.,

ZEPPLIN, M. and ELVEHJEM, C. A.: J. Nutr. **31**, 439 (1946).

248. ANDERSON, E. P., SMITH, J. K., ELVEHJEM, C. A. and PHILLIPS, P. H.: J. Nutr. **35**, 371 (1948).

249. SHAW, J. H.: J. Nutr. **38**, 275 (1949).

250. MCCLURE, F. J. and FOLK, J. E.: Proc. Soc. Exp. Biol. Med. **83**, 21 (1953).

251. JORDAN, H. V., FITZGERALD, R. J. and POOLE, W. C.: J. Dent. Res. **37**, 52 (1958).

252. ZEPPLIN, M., SMITH, J. K., PARSONS, H. T., PHILLIPS, P. H. and ELVEHJEM, C. A.: J. Nutr. **40**, 203 (1950).

253. STEINMAN, R. R., HARDINGE, M. G. and WOODS, R. W.: J. Dent. Res. **37**, 865, 874 (1958).

254. DALDERUP, L. M. and JANSEN, B. C. P.: Int. Rev. Vit. Res. **26**, 192 (1955).

255. DALDERUP, L. M. and JANSEN, B. C. P.: Int. Rev. Vit. Res. **26**, 199 (1955).

256. SHAW, J. H.: J. Nutr. **53**, 151 (1954).

257. GUSTAFSON, G., STELLING, E., ABRAMSON, E. and BRUNIUS, E.: Odontol. Tidskr. **61**, 386 (1953).

258. FITZGERALD, R. J.: Advances in Experimental Caries Research p. 187 (Washington D. C. 1955).

259. KITE, O. W., SHAW, J. H. and SOGNNAES, R. F.: J. Nutr. **42**, 89 (1950).

260. SHAW, J. H.: J. Nutr. **41**, 13 (1950).

261. GUSTAFSON, G., STELLING, E., ABRAMSON E. and BRUNIUS, E.: Odontol. Tidskr. **63**, 506 (1955).

262. KLAPPER, C. E. and VOLKER, J. F.: J. Dent. Res. **37**, 975 (1958).

263. BIXLER, D. and MÜHLER, J. C.: J. Dent. Res. **37**, 407 (1958).

264. SOGNNAES, R. F.: Amer. J. Orth. Oral Surg. (Oral Surg. Section) **27**, 552 (1941).

265. SHAW, J. H.: J. Dent. Res. **26**, 47 (1947).

266. HUNT, H. R. and HOPPERT, C. A.: J. Dent. Res. **27**, 553 (1948).

267. KAMRIN, B. B.: J. Dent. Res. **33**, 175 (1955).

268. KAMRIN, B. B.: J. Dent. Res. **33**, 824 (1955).

269. HUNT, H. R., HOPPERT, C. A. and ERWIN, W. G.: J. Dent. Res. **23**, 385 (1944).

270. DALDERUP, L. M.: J. Dent. Res. (in the press).

271. WISLOCKI, G. B. and SOGNNAES, R. F.: Amer. J. Anatomy **87**, 239 (1950).

272. MÉZL, Z.: Tijdschr. Tandhk. **58**, 614 (1951).

273. NIZEL, A. E. and HARRIS, R. S.: Arch. Biochem. **26**, 135 (1950).

274. SOGNNAES, R. F. and SHAW, J. H.: J. Nutr. **53**, 195 (1954).

275. SOGNNAES, R. F. and SHAW, J. H.: J. Nutr. **53**, 207 (1954).

276. NIZEL, A. E. and HARRIS, R. S.: J. Dent. Res. **34**, 513 (1955).

277. BÜTTNER, W., CREMER, H. D. and HARTUNG, W.: Dtsch. zahnärztl. Ztg. **12**, 541 (1957).

278. ROZEIK, F., CREMER, H. D. and HANNOVER, R.: ORCA, Proceedings of the 4th Congress, Odontol. revy **8**, 71 (1957).

279. JOHANSEN, E., STRAIN, W. and BARNARD, B.: J. Dent. Res. **37**, 33 (1958).

280. UNDERWOOD, E. J.: Trace Elements in Human and Animal Nutrition, (New York 1956).

281. SHAW, J. H.: Survey of the Literature of dental caries p. 415 (Washington 1952).

282. WYNN, W., HALDI, J., BENTLEY, K. D. and LAW, M. L.: J. Nutr. **58**, 325 (1956).

283. SOBEL, A. E. and HANOK, A.: J. Dent. Res. **37**, 631 (1958).

284. KEYES, P. H.: J. Dent. Res. **25**, 341 (1946).

285. NIZEL, A. E. and HARRIS, R. S.: J. Dent. Res. **37**, 35 (1958).

286. BARNARD, P. and JOHANSEN, E.: J. Dent. Res. **37**, 34 (1958).
287. BÜTTNER, W. and MÜHLER, J. C.: J. Dent. Res. **37**, 860 (1958).
288. DALDERUP, L. M.: J. Dent. Res. **38**, 1073 (1959).
289. CONSTANT, M. A., SIEVERT, H. W., PHILLIPS, P. H. and ELVEHJEM, C. A.: J. Nutr. **53**, 17 (1954).
290. CONSTANT, M. A., SIEVERT, H. W., PHILLIPS, P. H. and ELVEHJEM, C. A.: J. Nutr. **53**, 29 (1954).
291. MITCHELL, P. H.: A textbook of Biochemistry p. 533 (New York 1946).
292. MCCLURE, F. J.: J. Dent. Res. **27**, 34 (1948).
293. HEIN, J. W.: Advances in Experimental Caries Research, p. 197 (Washington D. C. 1955).
294. WYNN, W., HALDI, J., LAW, M. L. and BENTLEY, K. D.: J. Dent. Res. **37**, 33 (1958).
295. PARMA, C., DANEK, J. and HANUSOVA, N.: Cs. stom. **52**, 150 (1952) cited by de JONGE TH. E., Ned. Tijdschr. Gen. **98**, 1101 (1957).
296. IRVING, J. T. cited by PINDBORG, J. J.: Oral Surg., Oral Med., Oral Pathol. **6**, 780 (1953).
297. RYGH, O.: Bull. Soc. Chem. Biol. **31**, 1052 (1949).
298. DREIZEN, S., NIEDERMEYER, W., DREIZEN, J. G. and SPIES, T. D.: J. Dent. Res. **37**, 1149 (1958).
299. KRÜGER, B. J.: Univ. Queensland Papers **1**, 3 (1959).
300. GISH, C. W., MÜHLER, J. C. and HOWELL, C. L.: J. Dent. Res. **36**, 780 (1957).
301. MÜHLER, J. C. and DAY, H. G.: J. Amer. Dent. Ass. **41**, 528 (1950).
302. MÜHLER, J. C. and DAY, H. G.: J. Nutr. **44**, 413 (1951).
303. RADIKE, A. W. and MÜHLER, J. C.: J. Dent. Res. **32**, 807 (1953).
304. MÜHLER, J. C.: J. Dent. Res. **36**, 787 (1957).
305. RYGH, O.: Bull. Soc. Chem. Biol. **31**, 1403 (1949).

306. GEYER, C. F.: J. Dent. Res. **32**, 590 (1953).
307. HEIN, J. W. and WISOTSKY, J.: J. Dent. Res. **34**, 756 (1955).
308. WINIKER, M.: Proceedings of the 4th Congress ORCA, Odontol. revy **8**, 42 (1957).
309. MÜNCH, J.: Proceedings of the 4th Congress ORCA, Odontol. revy **8**, 52 (1957).
310. ADLER, P.: Proceedings of the 4th Congress ORCA, Odontol. revy **8**, 48 (1957).
311. SCHWARZ, K. cited in: Vitamin E and Selenium, part I and II, Nutr. Rev. **16**, 149 and 174 (1958).
312. HADJIMARKOS, D. M., STORVICK, C. A. and REMMERT, L. F.: J. Dent. Res. **31**, 505, 1952; J. Pediatr. **40**, 451 (1952).
313. HADJIMARKOS, D. M. and BONHORST, C. W.: J. Dent. Res. **37**, 971 (1958).
314. SMITH, M. I.: Publ. Health Rep. **51**, 1496 (1936).
315. WHEATCROFT, M. G., ENGLISH, J. A. and SLACK, C. A.: J. Dent. Res. **30**, 523 (1951).
316. MÜHLER, J. C. and SHAFER, W. G.: J. Dent. Res. **36**, 895 (1957).
317. ENGLISH, J. A.: J. Dent. Res. **28**, 172 (1949).
318. MÜHLER, J. C. and SHAFER, W. G.: Science **119**, 687 (1954).
319. MÜHLER, J. C., BIXLER, D. and SHAFER, W. G.: Proc. Soc. Exper. Biol. Med. **93**, 328 (1956).
320. WISOTZKY, J. and HEIN, J. W.: J. Dent. Res. **34**, 768 (1955).
321. GINN, J. T. and VOLKER, J. F.: Proc. Soc. Exper. Biol. Med. **57**, 189 (1944).
322. LEICESTER, H. M.: J. Dent. Res. **25**, 337 (1946).
323. WYNN, W. and HALDI, J.: J. Nutr. **54**, 285 (1954).
324. HALDI, J., WYNN, W. and SHAW, J. H.: J. Dent. Res. **37**, 33 (1958).
325. VENKATARAMANAN, K. and KRISHNASWANY, N.: Indian J. Med. Res.

37, 277 (1949); [Biol. Abstr. **24**, (9) 26236 (1950)].

326. WADHWANI, T. K.: J. Indian Inst. Sci. **36**, 64 (1954) see also Nutr. Abst. Rev. **24**, 656 (1954).

327. HEIN, J. W.: J. Dent. Rec. **32**, 654 (1953).

328. HEIN, J. W., QUIGLEY, G. A., and MARCUSSEN, H.: J. Dent. Res. **37**, 34 (1958).

329. RINEHART, J. F. and GREENBERG, L. D.: Amer. J. Clin. Nutr. **4**, 318 (1956).

330. STREAN, L. P., GILFILLIN, E. W. and EMERSON, G. A.: New York State Dent. J. **22**, 325 (1956).

331. STEINMAN, R. R., HEWES, C. G. and HARDINGE, M. G.: J. Dent. Res. **37**, 32 (1958).

332. BÜTTNER, W. and MÜHLER, J. C.: J. Dent. Res. **37**, 419 (1958).

333. CARTWRIGHT, K. L.: Nutr. Rev. **16**, 319 (1958).

334. MELLANBY, M.: Brit. Dent. J. march **1** (1937).

335. MELLANBY, H.: J. Dent. Res. **20**, 489 (1941).

336. HATTON, E. H. DODDS, A., HODGE, H. C. and FOSDICK, L. S.: J. Dent. Res. **24**, 283 (1945).

337. SHAW, J. H.: Proc. Soc. Exper. Biol. Med. **70**, 479 (1949).

338. GRANADOS, H., GLAVIND, J. and DAM, H.: Acta pathol. microbiol. Scand. **26**, 597 (1949).

339. ORLAND, F. J., HEMMENS, E. S. and HARRISON, R. W.: J. Dent. Res. **29**, 512 (1950).

340. GUSTAFSON, G., STELLING, E., ABRAMSON, E. and BRUNIUS, E.: Arch. Oral Biol. **1**, 42 (1959).

Author-Index

Subject Index

Zeitschrift für Ernährungswissenschaft

Journal of Nutritional Sciences – Journal des Sciences de la Nutrition

Unter Mitwirkung von

E. ABRAMSON-Stockholm, K. BERNHARD-Basel, J. BRÜGGEMANN-München, H. DAM-Kopenhagen, W. DROESE-München, A. HOCK-Berlin, J. KUPRIANOFF-Karlsruhe, W. LENKEIT-Göttingen, H. MALMROS-Lund, R. NICOLAYSEN-Oslo, L. SCHMID-Wien, und A. I. VIRTANEN-Helsinki

herausgegeben von

Prof. Dr. Dr. KONRAD LANG

Direktor des Physiologisch-chemischen Universitätsinstitutes Mainz

Begründet 1960. Erscheint zwanglos nach Bedarf. Vier Hefte bilden 1 Band. 1960 erschien Bd. 1. Die Hefte werden einzeln bei Erscheinen berechnet. Abonnementspreis pro Heft ca. DM 12,—, zuzügl. Porto. Einzelpreis ca. DM 14,—. 1961 erscheint Band 2 sowie Supplementum 1. Dieser Ergänzungsband (Aktuelle Probleme des Mineralstoffwechsels) wird zum Preise von DM 30,— (Abonnementspreis) bzw. DM 36,— (Einzelpreis) lieferbar sein.

In introducing the new publication, the editor refers to the impact of modern food processing on the science of nutrition and the new facets which food additives, agricultural chemicals, and the radiation treatment of foods add to nutritional research. Against this the refinement of research tools opens up new avenues in nutrition research.

This calls for a new medium of communications, says the editor, who is careful to point out that this new journal will try to be helpful to bring together information which ordinarily must be gleaned from a multitude of publications, and thus is not just another one.

It intends to bring publications in German, English and French.

Food Technology in Australia

Aus den ersten Heften:

H. DAM and M. CHRISTENSEN (Copenhagen), Alimentary production of gallstone in the golden hamster (VIII)

U.-M. NIEMI and P. ROINE (Helsinki), The effect of rapeseed oil on the thyroid function of rats.

P. ROINE, E. UKSILA, H. TEIR and J. RAPOLA (Helsinki), Histopathological changes in rats and pigs fed rapeseed oil.

G. VERDONK (Gand/Belgique), Athéromatose et diététique

G. VERDONK, A. VAN DER SCHUEREN, A. MOREAU et A. DE RUYTER (Gand/Belgique), Le travailleur et son alimentation en collectivité.

Probehefte stehen auf Wunsch zur Verfügung

Dr. DIETRICH STEINKOPFF VERLAG · DARMSTADT

Wissenschaftliche Veröffentlichungen der Deutschen Gesellschaft für Ernährung

Im Auftrage der Gesellschaft herausgegeben von Prof. Dr. Dr. *K. Lang*-Mainz

In dieser Reihe liegen bisher vor:

Band 1: **Die ernährungsphysiologischen Eigenschaften der Fette.** Vorträge und Diskussionen des 1. Symposions zu Mainz vom 30. 9. bis 1. 10.1957, unter der Leitung von Prof. Dr. Dr. *Konrad Lang*, Mainz. Mit einem Vorwort von Prof. Dr. *H. Kraut*, Dortmund. VIII, 190 Seiten mit 36 Abbildungen und 34 Tabellen. 1958. Karton. DM 35,—

Band 2: **Beiträge zum Antibiotika- und Eiweißproblem.** Hauptvorträge der 1. Wissenschaftlichen Arbeitstagung der Deutschen Gesellschaft für Ernährung zu Mainz vom 9. bis 11. April 1958, unter der Leitung von Prof. Dr. *Heinrich Kraut*, Dortmund. Mit einem Vorwort von Prof. Dr. Dr. *Konrad Lang*, Mainz. VII, 68 Seiten mit 3 Abb. und 11 Tab. 1959. Karton. DM 12,—

Band 3: **Arteriosklerose und Ernährung.** Vorträge und Diskussionen des 2. Symposions zu Bad Neuenahr vom 17.–18. Oktober 1958, unter der Leitung von Prof. Dr. *Hans Wilhelm Bansi*, Hamburg. Mit einem Vorwort von Prof. Dr. *Joachim Kühnau*, Hamburg. IX, 246 Seiten mit 80 Abbildungen und 28 Tabellen. 1959. Karton. DM 45,—

Band 4: **Akzeleration und Ernährung . Fettlösliche Wirkstoffe.** Hauptvorträge der 2. Wissenschaftlichen Arbeitstagung der Deutschen Gesellschaft für Ernährung zu Mainz vom 31. 3. bis 2. 4. 1959, unter der Leitung von Prof. Dr. *Joachim Kühnau*, Hamburg. Mit einem Vorwort von Prof. Dr. Dr. *Konrad Lang*, Mainz. VIII, 98 S. mit 19 Abb., 2 Schemata und 16 Tabellen. 1959. Karton. DM 19,—

Band 5: **Veränderungen der Nahrung durch industrielle und haushaltsmäßige Verarbeitung.** Vorträge und Diskussionen des 3. Symposions zu München vom 22.—23. Oktober 1959, unter der Leitung und mit einem Vorwort von Prof. Dr. Dr. *Konrad Lang*, Mainz. XI, 244 Seiten mit 40 Abb. 1 Schema und 52 Tabellen, 1960. Karton. DM 45,—

Band 6: **Kurort-Diät.** Vorträge und Diskussionen des 4. Symposions (in Gemeinschaft mit dem Deutschen Bäderverband e. V.) zu Bad Neuenahr vom 18. bis 19. März 1960, unter der Leitung von Prof. Dr. Dr. *Konrad Lang*, Mainz. Mit einem Vorwort von Prof. Dr. *J. Kühnau*, Hamburg. X, 116 Seiten, mit 2 Abb. und 12 Tab. 1961. Karton. DM 24,—

Band 7: **Hygienische Probleme bei Gewinnung, Verarbeitung und Vertrieb von Lebensmitteln.** Vorträge und Diskussionen des 5. Symposiums zu Mainz vom 7.–8. April 1960, unter der Leitung von Prof. Dr. *F. Klose*, Kiel. Etwa IX, 180 Seiten mit 38 Abbildungen und 7 Tabellen. 1961. Karton. ca. DM 35,—

Dr. DIETRICH STEINKOPFF VERLAG · DARMSTADT

Beiträge zur Ernährungswissenschaft

Herausgegeben von

W. DIEMAIR	J. KUPRIANOFF	K. LANG	C. H. MELLINGHOFF
Frankfurt/M.	Karlsruhe	Mainz	Wuppertal

Band 1

Biochemie der Ernährung

Von Prof. Dr. Dr. KONRAD LANG

Direktor des Physiologisch-chemischen Universitätsinstituts Mainz

XVI, 412 Seiten mit 9 Abb., 24 Schemata und 214 Tabellen, 1957. Ganzln. DM 54,—

This is the first volume of an intended new series entitled "Beiträge zur Ernährungswissenschaft" with contributions both from medicine, physiology, physiological chemistry, chemistry, and from veterinary and engineering sciences. The editor has made it his aim to produce a work that is concise, clear and stimulative of interest. The present volumed ealing with the carbohydrates, fats, proteins, cholesterin, mineral substances and vitamins, is a promising start with a multitude of information of value to the internist.

Acta medica Scandinavica

This excellent summary is the first in a series devoted to foods and nutrition... The work is well printed and very readable... Since later volumes are to be devoted to common foodstuffs, human nutrition, and nutritional diseases, this introductory volume should provide an excellent starting point for those who wish to read the series.

Archives of Biochemistry and Biophysics

Band 2

Der Diabetes mellitus als Volkskrankheit und seine Beziehung zur Ernährung

Von Prof. Dr. Dr. ERNST-GÜNTHER SCHENCK-Starnberg (Obb.)
und Prof. Dr. C. H. MELLINGHOFF-Wuppertal

XI, 310 Seiten mit 10 Abbildungen und 60 Tabellen. 1960. Ganzleinen DM 54,—

This is a solid and comprehensive work, liberally sprinkled with references to investigations and surveys in Germany and other countries... Clinical aspects, including the complications which may arise and finally cause death, and forms of treatment are of course considered at length.

Nutrition Abstracts and Reviews

Dr. DIETRICH STEINKOPFF VERLAG · DARMSTADT

Beiträge zur Ernährungswissenschaft

Band 3 *Strahlenkonservierung und Kontamination von Lebensmitteln*

Von Prof. Dr. JOHANN KUPRIANOFF
Direktor der Bundesforschungsanstalt für Lebensmittelfrischhaltung Karlsruhe

und Prof. Dr. Dr. KONRAD LANG
Direktor des Physiologisch-chemischen Instituts der Universität Mainz

XVI, 297 Seiten mit 40 Abbildungen, 1 Schema und 145 Tabellen, 1960.
Ganzleinen DM 64,—

This is the first German monography dealing with this important subject. Basing on the experiences of two German scientists during a trip through the USA, the book gives a comprehensive survey on international research of today.
Well printed with 35 figures and 145 schedules, the index of 788 numbers is to be mentioned seperately. Thus the book will soon become an important hand-book and will be of great use to anyone interested in these special questions of nutrition.

Band 4 *Die experimentelle diätetische Lebernekrose*

Von Dr. Dr. KLAUS STRUNZ und Prof. Dr. ANDREAS HOCK
Institut für Tierernährungslehre der Humboldt-Universität Berlin

XII, 124 Seiten mit 12 Tabellen. 1960. Ganzleinen DM 28,—

This small book is devoted solely to an analysis of various diets used in the production of hepatic necrosis . . . This volume will be useful to anyone interested in necrogenic diets in experimental animals. The various factors in these diets are thoroughly reviewed, and adequate references are presented.
American Journal of Digestive Diseases

Band 5 *Die Vitamine in der Diät- und Küchenpraxis*

Von Prof. Dr. FRITZ HEEPE
Oberarzt der Medizinischen Klinik und Poliklinik der Universität Münster

Mit einem Geleitwort von Prof. Dr. W. H. HAUSS, Münster (Westf.)
Direktor der Medizinischen Klinik und Poliklinik der Universität Münster

XIII, 232 Seiten mit 80 Tabellen und 185 Rezeptbeispielen. 1961.
Ganzleinen DM 44,—

Dr. DIETRICH STEINKOPFF VERLAG · DARMSTADT